EXAMINATION REVIEW FOR ULTRASOUND

SONOGRAPHIC PRINCIPLES & INSTRUMENTATION (SPI)

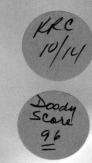

EXAMINATION REVIEW FOR ULTRASOUND

SONOGRAPHIC PRINCIPLES & INSTRUMENTATION (SPI)

Steven M. Penny, BS, RT(R), RDMS
Medical Sonography Lead Instructor
Health Sciences Department
Johnston Community College
Smithfield, North Carolina

Traci B. Fox, MS, RT(R), RDMS, RVT
Instructor and Clinical Coordinator, DMS Program
Department of Radiologic Sciences
Jefferson School of Health Professions
Thomas Jefferson University
Philadelphia, Pennsylvania

Cathy Herring Godwin, MEd, RT(R), RDMS, RDCS, RVT
Director of Sonography Programs
Health Sciences Department
Johnston Community College
Smithfield, North Carolina

Contributor: B. Dwight Gunter BS, RDMS
Program Director
Department of Diagnostic Medical Sonography
Sanford-Brown College
Atlanta, Georgia

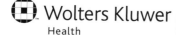 Wolters Kluwer | Lippincott Williams & Wilkins
Health

Philadelphia · Baltimore · New York · London
Buenos Aires · Hong Kong · Sydney · Tokyo

Acquisitions Editor: Peter Sabatini
Product Director: Tanya M. Martin
Associate Product Manager: Erin M. Cosyn
Marketing Manager: Shauna Kelley
Compositor: MPS Limited, a Macmillan Company

Two Commerce Square
2001 Market Street
Philadelphia, PA 19103 USA
LWW.com

Printed in China

Library of Congress Cataloging-in-Publication Data

Penny, Steven M.
Examination review for ultrasound: sonographic principles & instrumentation (SPI)/
Steven M. Penny, Traci B. Fox, Cathy Herring Godwin.
    p. ; cm.
  Includes bibliographical references and index.
  ISBN 978-1-60831-137-8
  1. Diagnostic imaging—Examinations, questions, etc. I. Fox, Traci B.
  II. Godwin, Cathy Herring. III. Title.
  [DNLM: 1. Ultrasonography–methods—Examination Questions.
  2. Ultrasonography—instrumentation—Examination Questions. WN 18.2]
  RC78.7.U4P36 2011
  616.07'543076–dc22

                                                            2010044287

To purchase additional copies of this book, call our customer service department at (800) 638-3030 or fax orders to (301) 223-2320. International customers should call (301) 223-2300.

DEDICATION

To my father and mother, both of whom have made countless sacrifices throughout their lives in order for me to become the man and father I am today. Without your love and devotion and your willingness to put my needs before your own, I would never have appreciated my own potential. Your example has shown me that my life should be lived in continual pursuance of His will, not my own. I will be forever thankful that you were chosen to be my parents, and yet eternally undeserving.

S.M.P

To Thresa, my rock, my spirit, and my sounding board, your indomitable patience and support made it possible for me to survive not only this project but all my others as well.

T.B.F.

To my three wonderful sons, Sonny Jr., Corey, and Chris, you are my inspiration and my life. And to my mother and father, Louis and Linda Herring, you are my strength and vision. With God, all things are possible.

C.H.G.

PREFACE

Sonography is a multifaceted and unique profession. It consists of a small community of clinical and imaging specialists. As sonographers we not only play a crucial role in the health management of our patients, but we pride ourselves in the fact that we have the ability to perform distinctive, influential patient care. Sonographers do not simply take pictures but rather perform investigative imaging. We must be malleable, subsequently prepared to adjust each sonographic study based on clinical history and unpredictable sonographic findings. The opportunity to utilize critical thinking is a unique assignment for the sonographer.

With such a distinctive role comes a distinctive obligation. We cannot merely perform the examination without a thought beyond the task at hand. We must have a fundamental appreciation of how our images are created, and thus how sound can be used to produce an image of the human body. Absolute patient care demands that all sonographers not only have the ability to obtain a diagnostic image but also have the ability to understand how that image is shaped. Knowledgeable practitioners realize both the limitation and growing potential for sonography. Although the use of ultrasound on human tissue has not yet been definitively proven to cause any sustainable biologic effects at diagnostic ranges, we must still practice in a way respectful and mindful to the science behind the image.

OBJECTIVE

Our responsibility in advancing the diagnostic implications of sonography is apparent, but more importantly, we must be capable of providing consistent high-quality patient care. Standardized testing through credential granting organizations such as the American Registry for Diagnostic Medical Sonography (ARDMS) affords our profession a means of necessitating competency, a competency that all patients not only expect but deserve. Accordingly, the objective of *Examination Review for Ultrasound: Sonographic Principles & Instrumentation (SPI)* is to provide a straightforward comprehensive review in sonographic physics.

ORGANIZATION

The ARDMS introduced the newest installment of its sonographic physics examination in the spring of 2009 with the release of the Sonographic Principles and Instrumentation (SPI) examination. The SPI examination must be taken by all specialties, including cardiac, vascular, and general concentrations, as part of becoming a registered sonographer. The newest version (2010) of the SPI includes six general themes: patient care, physics principles, ultrasound transducers, display modes, Doppler instrumentation and hemodynamics, and quality assurance. Accordingly, this text is presented in this fashion.

The structure of each chapter is similar. Key terms provided at the beginning of each chapter act as a study aid. In the back of the book, the student will find a glossary of all the key terms mentioned throughout the book for easy reference. Also, uncomplicated narrative is offered and further reinforced by summary tables and high-quality figures. Basic chapter review questions are offered at the end of each chapter as well. These questions will allow for an assessment of one's grasp of the chapter's content. An answer key is offered in the back of the book.

ADDITIONAL RESOURCES

The registry review does not end with the conclusion of this book. Because computer-based testing has become the principal device for administering certification examinations, we have supplied the student with an opportunity to take a computer-based mock exam. A registry review examination is provided online to those who purchase this book. By accessing the thePoint at **thepoint.lww.com/product/isbn/9781608311378**, the reader will have the opportunity to take computer-based examinations with more intense "registry-like" questions. Other instructor and student resources and review materials can be found online: the faculty resource center includes an image bank, chapter outlines, PowerPoint presentations, and the mock exams. The student resource center includes the mock exam and image bank.

FINAL NOTE

For many, fear proliferates with the mere mention of the word "physics." This book is unique. It is not written by physicists, physicians, or nonimaging professionals. It is matchless because it is written by sonographers for sonographers. The narrative is easy to read and understand. It provides just enough information to not overwhelm the reader, while at the same time reinforcing fundamental principles with a straightforward approach.

The material contained is deliberately not exhaustive so that the review is not hindered by an overwhelming amount of statistics, formulas, and superfluous information. Therefore, there are several uses of this book that are inherent in its arrangement. It is certainly suitable for implementation in the classroom environment. Instructors offering registry review classes will benefit considerably by adopting this text. The structure will provide the educator the opportunity to assign a review of one topic at a time, while affording the recognition and correction of subject matter weaknesses. It should also be helpful to individuals who have completed a formal educational program and who need a realistic gauge of material mastery before attempting the examination. Lastly, for those who must take the examination after years of clinical practice in order to obtain additional certification, this book is written to provide the clear-cut review of sonographic physics that you want. Whether you use this book to refresh or reinforce your understanding of sonographic physics, may the knowledge that you acquire from its pages not only be maintained through the examination period, but may it also be exploited in your daily practice as a registered sonographer.

Steven M. Penny

REVIEWERS

RENATO M. AGUSTIN, MD, RDMS, RVT
Program Director
Diagnostic Medical Sonography Department
Sanford-Brown College
Cleveland, OH

SHARLETTE ANDERSON, MHS, RDMS, RVT, RDCS
Clinical Coordinator/Instructor
DMU Program
University of Missouri
Columbia, MO

TERRENCE D. CASE, EDM, RVT, FSVU
Program Director, Assistant Professor
Cardiovascular Sonography Program
Nova Southeastern University
Fort Lauderdale, FL

B. DWIGHT GUNTER, BS, RDMS
Program Director
Diagnostic Medical Sonography Department
Sanford-Brown College
Atlanta, GA

BETTYE G. WILSON, MAEd, RT(R)(CT) ARRT, RDMS, FASRT
Associate Professor Emerita
School of Health Professions
University of Alabama at Birmingham
Birmingham, AL

ACKNOWLEDGMENTS

This book would not be possible without the love and support of my wife Lisa. The happiness that she and our children, Devin and Reagan, freely share with me fuels my accomplishments and brightens every moment of my life. Credit again should be given to Cathy Herring Godwin for her patience and guidance throughout my career as a sonographer. I would also like to acknowledge Traci B. Fox for stepping up and offering, with unbridled confidence, her knowledge in ultrasound physics at the ideal time. Once more, I owe my acquisition editor Peter Sabatini a vast amount of gratitude for having faith in my abilities as an author. Recognition must be given to Erin M. Cosyn at LWW as well for her excellent direction throughout this project. Lastly, to all of my students, both past and present, thank you for teaching me more about sonography than I ever thought I would know.

S.M.P.

I would like to thank Steven M. Penny for inviting me along on this journey. I would also like to thank my department chair, Fran Gilman, my program director Dr Nandu Rawool, my fellow faculty, and my family for all their support. In addition, many thanks to Dr Barry Goldberg, Dr Flemming Forsberg, and Larry Waldroup from the Jefferson Ultrasound Research and Education Institute, Drs Carl Rubin and Jason Sagerman from Aria Health, and all my fellow sonographers who have always supported my endeavors.

T.B.F.

Thank you to all of the sonographers I've been blessed to know over the years. And to my coworkers, Steven M. Penny and Catherine Rominski, you are the best friends anyone could work with.

C.H.G.

CONTENTS

CHAPTER 1

Physics Principles

INTRODUCTION

This chapter focuses on units of measurement and the properties of sound. The purpose of this chapter is to provide a foundation for more complex material found in the following chapters.

KEY TERMS

absorption—the conversion of sound energy to heat

acoustic speckle—the interference pattern caused by scatterers that produces the granular appearance of tissue on a sonographic image

amplitude—the maximum or minimum deviation of an acoustic variable from the average value of that variable; the strength of the reflector

attenuation—a decrease in the amplitude, power, and intensity of the sound beam as sound travels through tissue

1

attenuation coefficient—the rate at which sound is attenuated per unit depth

axial resolution—the ability to accurately identify reflectors that are arranged parallel to the ultrasound beam

backscatter—scattered sound waves that make their way back to the transducer and produce an image on the display

compression—an area in the sound wave where the molecules are pushed closer together

continuous wave—sound that is continuously transmitted

damping—the process of reducing the number of cycles of each pulse in order to improve axial resolution

decibels (dB)—a unit that establishes a relationship or comparison between two values of power or intensity

density—mass per unit volume

directly related—relationship that implies that if one variable decreases, the other also decreases or if one variable increases, the other also increases

distance—how far apart objects are

duty factor—the percentage of time that sound is actually being produced

elasticity—see key term stiffness

frequency—the number of cycles per second

hydrophone—a device used to measure output intensity of the transducer

impedance—the resistance to the propagation of sound through a medium

inertia—Newton's principle that states that an object at rest stays at rest and an object in motion stays in motion, unless acted on by an outside force

intensity—the power of the wave divided by the area over which it is spread; the energy per unit area

intensity reflection coefficient—the percentage of sound reflected at an interface

intensity transmission coefficient—the percentage of sound transmitted at an interface

interface—the dividing line between two different media

inversely related—relationship that implies that if one variable decreases, the other increases or if one variable increases, the other decreases

longitudinal waves—the molecules of the medium vibrate back and forth in the same direction that the wave is traveling

medium—any form of matter: solid, liquid, or gas

nonspecular reflectors—reflectors that are smaller than the wavelength of the incident beam

normal incidence—angle of incidence is 90° to the interface

oblique incidence—angle of incidence is lesser than or greater than 90° to the interface

parameter—a measurable quantity

particle motion—the movement of molecules due to propagating sound energy

path length—distance to the reflector

period—the time it takes for one cycle to occur

piezoelectric materials—a material that generates electricity when pressure is applied to it, and one that changes shape when electricity is applied to it; also referred to as the element

power—the rate at which work is performed or energy is transmitted

pressure—force per unit area or the concentration of force

propagate—to transmit through a medium

propagation speed—the speed at which a sound wave travels through a medium

pulse duration—the time during which the sound is actually being transmitted; the "on" time

pulse repetition frequency—the number of pulses of sound produced in 1 second

pulse repetition period—the time taken for a pulse to occur

pulsed wave—sound that is sent out in pulses

rarefaction—an area in the sound wave where the molecules are spread wider apart

Rayleigh scatterers—very small reflectors

reflection—the echo; part of sound that returns from an interface

refraction—change in direction of the transmitted sound beam that occurs with oblique incidence and dissimilar propagation speeds

scattering—the phenomenon that occurs when sound waves are forced to deviate from a straight path secondary to changes within the medium

Snell's law—used to describe the angle of transmission at an interface based on the angle of incidence and the propagation speeds of the two media

sound—a traveling variation in pressure

spatial pulse length—the length of a pulse

specular reflections—reflections that occur when the sound impinges upon a large, smooth reflector at a 90° angle

stiffness—the ability of an object to resist compression and relates to the hardness of a medium

total attenuation—the total amount of sound (in dB) that has been attenuated at a given depth

transverse waves—type of wave in which the molecules in a medium vibrate at 90° to the direction of travel

wavelength—the length of a single cycle of sound

FUNDAMENTALS AND UNITS OF MEASUREMENTS

Fundamentals

The sonographer should be aware of the metric prefixes, their symbols, and their meaning (Table 1-1). Also, since ultrasound deals with small units of measurement, sonographers must have a fundamental appreciation for fractions of whole numbers and their symbols (Table 1-2). Understanding the conversion of units is also significant. Figure 1-1 summarizes how to convert units.

BASICS OF SOUND

What Is Sound?

Sound is a form of energy. It is a pressure wave, created by a mechanical action, and is therefore called a mechanical wave. Sound is produced when a vibrating source causes the molecules of a **medium** to move back and forth. This backward and forward movement of the molecules creates waves of sound energy that travel, or **propagate**, through the medium. A medium is

FIGURE 1-1 Conversion of units. When the metric prefix gets larger (e.g., mL to L, or mm to m), the number in front of the prefix gets smaller. To convert to a larger prefix, the decimal point will move to the left. (Notice that "larger" and "left" both begin with an "L.") In this example, a conversion is made from 1000 mm to meters. The prefix is getting larger, so the decimal point moves to the left. How much does one move the decimal point? The scientific notation for milli- is 10^{-3}, so the decimal point moves three places to the left. Therefore, 1000 mm is equal to 1 m. Converting from larger to smaller units would be the same idea, except the decimal point moves to the right.

TABLE 1-1	Metric whole numbers.		
Prefix	Symbol	Meaning	Value
Giga	G	Billion	10^9
Mega	M	Million	10^6
Kilo	k	Thousand	10^3
Hecto	h	Hundred	10^2
Deca	da	Ten	10^1

TABLE 1-2	Fractions of whole numbers.		
Prefix	Symbol	Meaning	Value
Nano	n	Billionth	10^{-9}
Micro	μ	Millionth	10^{-6}
Milli	m	Thousandth	10^{-3}
Centi	c	Hundredth	10^{-2}
Deci	d	Tenth	10^{-1}

1000. mm ⟶ 1.000 m

FIGURE 1-2 Example of longitudinal waves. If a gust of wind blows over a field of tall grass, the stalks bend back and forth in the same direction the wind is blowing **(A)**. If another gust of wind blows by, the longitudinal movement is repeated. The energy is traveling in the form of a longitudinal wave **(B)**. The movement of the grass is in the same direction parallel to the movement of the wave.

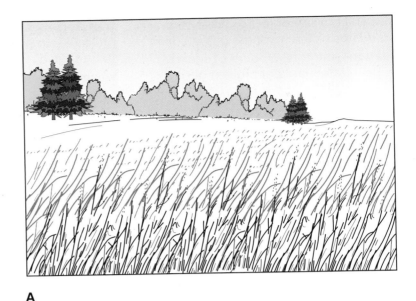

A

B

Longitudinal

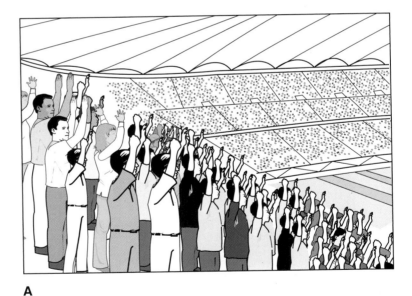

A

Transverse

B

FIGURE 1-3 Example of transverse waves. When spectators in a stadium do "the wave," we are experiencing a transverse wave. The arms of the spectators move up and down at 90° to the direction of travel, which is horizontally around the stadium **(A)**. The arms of the spectators do not move in the same direction as the wave is moving, but rather it moves in a direction perpendicular to the travel of the wave **(B)**.

TABLE 1-3 The three primary acoustic variables, their definitions, and their units.		
Acoustic Variable	**Definition**	**Units**
Pressure	Force per unit area or the concentration of force	Pascals (Pa) or pounds per square inch (lb/in^2)
Density	Mass per unit volume	Kilograms per centimeter cubed (kg/cm^3)
Distance	How far apart objects are	Feet, inches, centimeters, or miles

any form of matter: solid, liquid, or gas. Sound requires a medium in which to propagate; therefore, it cannot travel in a vacuum.

When sound energy propagates through a medium, it does so in **longitudinal waves**, meaning that the molecules of the medium vibrate back and forth in the same direction that the wave is traveling (Figure 1-2). In summary, sound is a mechanical, longitudinal wave. Longitudinal waves should not be confused with **transverse waves** where molecules in a medium vibrate at 90° to the direction of the traveling wave (Figure 1-3).

Acoustic Variables

Acoustic variables are changes that occur within a medium as a result of sound traveling through that medium. The three primary acoustic variables are **pressure**, **density**, and **distance** (Table 1-3). As stated in the previous section, when sound energy propagates through a medium, it causes the molecules to move back and forth. Each back and forth movement completes one wave or one cycle of movement. Each cycle consists of two parts: a **compression**, where the molecules are pushed closer together, and a **rarefaction**, where they are spread wider apart (Figure 1-4). The molecules, as they are squeezed together and separated, cause changes in the pressure

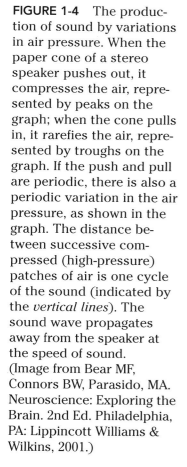

FIGURE 1-4 The production of sound by variations in air pressure. When the paper cone of a stereo speaker pushes out, it compresses the air, represented by peaks on the graph; when the cone pulls in, it rarefies the air, represented by troughs on the graph. If the push and pull are periodic, there is also a periodic variation in the air pressure, as shown in the graph. The distance between successive compressed (high-pressure) patches of air is one cycle of the sound (indicated by the *vertical lines*). The sound wave propagates away from the speaker at the speed of sound. (Image from Bear MF, Connors BW, Parasido, MA. Neuroscience: Exploring the Brain. 2nd Ed. Philadelphia, PA: Lippincott Williams & Wilkins, 2001.)

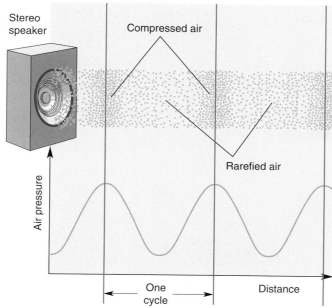

within the medium. Similarly, molecules undergoing compression and rarefaction show variations in density. Density is defined as mass per unit volume. This movement of molecules, or **particle motion**, is due to propagating sound energy. Distance is defined as how far apart objects are, and it is the measurement of particle motion. Distance may also be referred to as vibration or displacement.

PARAMETERS OF SOUND

A **parameter** is a measurable quantity. As this chapter progresses, the relationship that parameters of sound have with each other is discussed. Parameters may be described as **directly related** (directly proportional) or **inversely related** (inversely proportional) to each other. They are directly related when, if one parameter decreases, the other also decreases. Parameters are inversely related when one variable decreases, the other increases. Sound waves have several parameters that may be utilized to describe them. Parameters of sound waves include the **period**, **frequency**, **amplitude**, **power**, **intensity**, **propagation speed**, and **wavelength**.

Period and Frequency

Period (T) is defined as the time it takes for one cycle to occur (Figure 1-5). Since period is measured in time units, it is most often described in microseconds (μs), or one millionth of a second (Table 1-4). Frequency (f) is defined as the number of cycles per second (Figure 1-6). Frequency is measured in hertz (Hz), kilohertz (kHz), or megahertz (MHz) (Table 1-5). Frequency and period are inversely related. Therefore, as frequency increases, the period decreases, and as frequency decreases, the period increases (Table 1-6). Their relationship is also said to be reciprocal (Tables 1-7 and 1-8). When two reciprocals are multiplied together, the product is 1. Consequently, period multiplied by frequency equals 1.

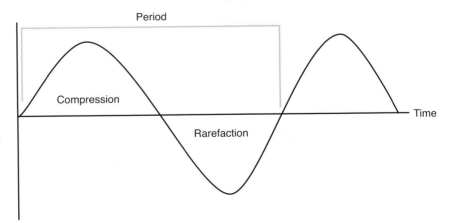

FIGURE 1-5 Period. Period is defined as the time it takes for one cycle to occur. One cycle consists of one compression and one rarefaction.

TABLE 1-4	Period.	
Term	**Definition**	**Units**
Period	The time it takes for one cycle to occur	Microseconds (μs), one millionth of a second

FIGURE 1-6 Frequency. Frequency is defined as the number of cycles per second.

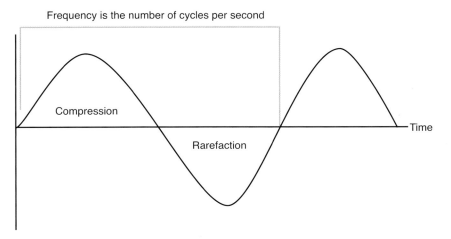

T A B L E 1 - 5 Frequency.		
Term	**Definition**	**Units**
Frequency	The number of cycles per second	Hertz (Hz), kilohertz (kHz), or megahertz (MHz)

T A B L E 1 - 6 The relationship between frequency and period.
Relationship
↑ Frequency ↓ Period
↓ Frequency ↑ Period

T A B L E 1 - 7 Formula for period.
Formula
$\text{Period} = \dfrac{1}{\text{Frequency}}$
$T = \dfrac{1}{f}$

T A B L E 1 - 8 Formula for frequency.
Formula
$\text{Frequency} = \dfrac{\text{Propagation speed}}{\text{Wavelength}}$
$f = \dfrac{c}{\lambda}$

Propagation Speed

Propagation speed (c) is defined as the speed at which a sound wave travels through a medium (Table 1-9). All sound, regardless of its frequency, travels at the same speed through any particular medium. Therefore, a 20-Hz sound wave and a 20-MHz sound wave travel at the same speed in a given medium

TABLE 1-9 Propagation speed.		
Term	**Definition**	**Units**
Propagation speed	The speed through which a sound wave travels through a medium	Meters per second (m/s) or millimeters per microsecond (mm/µs)

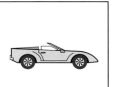 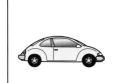 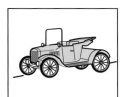

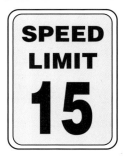

FIGURE 1-7 Propagation speed. All sound, regardless of its frequency, travels at the same speed through any particular medium. The maximum speed limit is 15 mph regardless of what car you drive.

(Figure 1-7). Propagation speeds tend to be the fastest in solids, such as bone, and slowest in gases or gas-containing structures, such as the lungs (Table 1-10). In the body, sound travels at slightly different speeds through the various organs and tissues. The units for propagation speed are meters per second (m/s) or millimeters per microsecond (mm/µs). The average speed of sound in all soft tissue is considered to be 1540 m/s or 1.54 mm/µs. This number was derived by averaging all of the actual propagation speeds of the tissues in the body.

The propagation speed of sound in a medium is influenced by two properties: the **stiffness** (**elasticity**) and the density (**inertia**) of the medium (Table 1-11). Stiffness is defined as the ability of an object to resist compression and relates to the hardness of a medium. Stiffness and propagation speed are directly related: the stiffer the medium, the faster the propagation speed. Conversely, density, which can be defined as the amount of mass in an object, is inversely related to propagation speed. As the density of a

TABLE 1-10 A list of media and their propagation speeds.	
Medium	**Propagation Speed**
Air	330 m/s
Lungs	660 m/s
Water	1480 m/s
Soft tissue	1540 m/s (average)
Liver	1555 m/s
Blood	1560 m/s
Bone	4080 m/s

T A B L E **1 - 1 1** The relationship among stiffness, density, and propagation speed.
Relationship
↑ Stiffness ↑ Propagation speed
↑ Density ↓ Propagation speed

T A B L E **1 - 1 2** Formula for propagation speed.
Formula
$\text{Propagation speed} = \dfrac{\text{Elasticity}}{\text{Density}}$
$c = \dfrac{e}{\rho \ (\text{rho})}$

medium increases, the propagation speed decreases (Table 1-12). For example, lead is an extremely dense metal; however, pure lead is not very stiff, as it is quite flexible and therefore bends easily. Subsequently, the propagation speed in lead is very slow. On the contrary, compact bone is not as dense as lead, but is much stiffer, resulting in a much faster propagation speed.

Wavelength

The length of a single cycle of sound is called the wavelength (λ). It is the distance from the beginning of a cycle to the end of that cycle (Figure 1-8). Waves can be of any length, from several miles in some ocean waves to a few millimeters, as found in diagnostic ultrasound waves. In clinical imaging, the wavelengths measure between 0.1 and 0.8 mm (Table 1-13). Like period, wavelength and frequency are inversely related (Table 1-14). If frequency increases, wavelength decreases and vice versa. However, the wavelength of a sound wave is also influenced by the propagation speed of the medium in which it is traveling. The faster the propagation speed, the longer the wavelength. So, using our previous sample media, the wavelength of a given frequency would be very short in lead but much longer in bone. In diagnostic

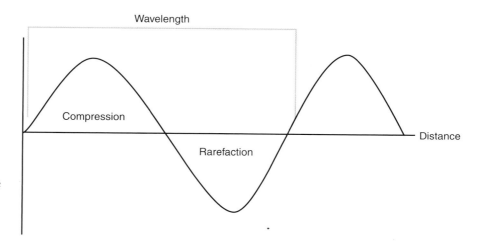

FIGURE 1-8 Wavelength. Wavelength is the distance from the beginning of a cycle to the end of that cycle.

TABLE 1-13	Wavelength.	
Term	**Definition**	**Units**
Wavelength	The distance over which one cycle occurs, or the distance from the beginning of one cycle to the end of that same cycle	Millimeters (mm)

TABLE 1-14 The relationship between wavelength and frequency.
Relationship
↑ Frequency ↓ Wavelength
↓ Frequency ↑ Wavelength

TABLE 1-15 Formula for wavelength.
Formula
$\text{Wavelength} = \dfrac{\text{Propagation speed}}{\text{Frequency}}$
$\lambda = \dfrac{c}{f}$

imaging, because the average propagation speed of sound in soft tissue is treated as a constant of 1540 m/s, any change in the wavelength would be related only to changes in the frequency. Wavelength is in essence equal to the propagation speed divided by the frequency $\lambda = c/f$ where $c = 1540$ m/s or 1.54 mm/μs (Table 1-15). It is important to note that the wavelength of a 1- and 2-MHz transducer is 1.54 and 0.77 mm, respectively.

Amplitude, Power, and Intensity

Amplitude, power, and intensity all relate to the size or strength of the sound wave (Tables 1-16 and 1-17). All three of these decrease as sound travels through a medium. Amplitude (A) is defined as the maximum or minimum deviation of an acoustic variable from the average value of that variable (Figure 1-9). For example, on a road trip, an average velocity may be 55 mph, but occasional increases of speed of up to 60 mph or decreases of speed down to 50 mph may occur. In this situation, the amplitude would be 5 mph, because that is the maximum and minimum variation from the average velocity. Note that the amplitude is not the difference between the maximum and the minimum extremes. As sound propagates through a medium, the acoustic variables (distance, density, and pressure) will vary, and therefore, they may increase or decrease. The amplitude of these changes can be measured. When amplitude is discussed in ultrasound physics, it is commonly the pressure amplitude that is being referenced. The units of amplitude are Pascals (Pa).

Power (P) is defined as the rate at which work is performed or energy is transmitted. As a sound wave travels through the body, it loses some of its energy. Therefore, power decreases as the sound wave moves through the body. The power of a sound wave is typically described in units of watts (W) or

T A B L E 1 - 1 6 Sound wave strength descriptor and their units.

Sound Wave Strength Descriptor	Definition	Units
Amplitude	The maximum value or minimum value of an acoustic variable minus the equilibrium value of that variable; the strength of the reflector	Pascals (Pa)
Power	The rate at which work is performed or energy is transmitted. As a sound wave travels through the body, it loses some amount of energy	Watts (W) or milliwatts (mW)
Intensity	The amount or degree of strength of sound per unit area or the energy per unit area	Units of watts per centimeter (W/cm) or watts per centimeter squared (W/cm^2)

T A B L E 1 - 1 7 The relationships of the sound wave strength descriptors.

Relationship
Power is proportional to amplitude squared
Power decreases as amplitude decreases
Intensity is proportional both to power and to amplitude squared

milliwatts (mW). Power is proportional to the amplitude squared (Table 1-18). Therefore, if the amplitude doubles, the power quadruples.

The intensity (I) of a sound wave is defined as the power of the wave divided by the area (a) over which it is spread, or the energy per unit area (Table 1-19). Intensity is proportional both to power ($I \propto P$) and to amplitude squared ($I \propto A^2$). Intensity is measured in units of watts per centimeter squared (W/cm^2) or milliwatts per centimeter squared (mW/cm^2). Intensities typically range from 0.01 to 100 mW/cm^2 for diagnostic ultrasound. Intensity is discussed in more detail later in this chapter (See section "More about Intensity").

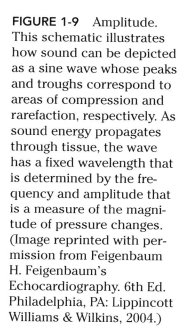

FIGURE 1-9 Amplitude. This schematic illustrates how sound can be depicted as a sine wave whose peaks and troughs correspond to areas of compression and rarefaction, respectively. As sound energy propagates through tissue, the wave has a fixed wavelength that is determined by the frequency and amplitude that is a measure of the magnitude of pressure changes. (Image reprinted with permission from Feigenbaum H. Feigenbaum's Echocardiography. 6th Ed. Philadelphia, PA: Lippincott Williams & Wilkins, 2004.)

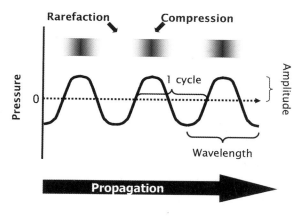

TABLE 1-18 Relationship of power and amplitude.
Relationship
$P \propto A^2$

TABLE 1-19 Formula for intensity.
Formula
$I = \dfrac{\text{Power (W)}}{\text{Area (cm}^2)}$

TABLE 1-20 Formula for impedance.
Formula
$z = \rho c$

Impedance

Any medium through which sound is traveling will offer some amount of resistance to the sound. For example, some of us can run fairly quickly on dry land. But trying to run at the same speed in 3 ft of water would be quite challenging. The water resists or impedes our movement. This resistance to the propagation of sound through a medium is called **impedance** (z). The amount of impedance depends on the density (ρ) and the propagation speed (c) of the medium. Keep in mind that the density and stiffness are the controlling factors of propagation speed. Impedance is measured in units called Rayls. Rayls are the product of the density of the medium and the propagation speed of sound in the medium (Table 1-20).

There are slight variations in the density of the various tissues in the body just as there are slight variations in the propagation speed. Recall that 1540 m/s is used as the *average* speed of sound in all soft tissue. As a result, many of the tissues will have different impedance values. It is these variations in impedance that help create reflections at the **interface** between adjacent tissues. Assuming the beam strikes the interface at a 90° angle and there exists a large impedance difference between two tissues, there will be a strong **reflection** and a well-defined boundary displayed on the imaging screen. If the impedance difference between two media is more subtle, there will be a weaker reflection. If the impedances are the same, no reflection occurs.

CONTINUOUS WAVE ULTRASOUND

Thus far in this chapter, we have been describing properties of all sound waves, which certainly apply to ultrasound waves as well. Sound that is continuously transmitted is termed **continuous wave** (CW) sound. We cannot image using CW ultrasound, though it is often employed for Doppler studies.

PULSE–ECHO TECHNIQUE AND PARAMETERS OF PULSED SOUND

Pulse–Echo Technique

In order for an image to be created using sound, the sound waves must not only be sent into the body, but the sound returning from the body must be timed to determine the reflector's distance from the transducer; this describes the pulse–echo technique (Figure 1-10). After a pulse is sent out, the machine listens for the sound to come back and calculates how long it takes for the pulse to come back to the transducer. As a result of waiting for the pulse of sound to come back and timing its travel, the machine is able to plot the location of the reflectors on the display.

Transducers have material within them that, when electronically stimulated, produces ultrasound waves. These are referred to as **piezoelectric materials** (PZT) and most likely consist of some form of lead zirconate titanate. PZT materials operate according to the principle of piezoelectricity, which states that pressure is created when voltage is applied to the material and electricity is created when a pressure is applied to the material (Figure 1-11). *Piezo* literally means to squeeze or press. Within the transducer, the element is electronically stimulated or stressed, which results in

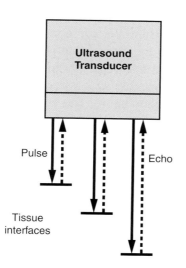

FIGURE 1-10   Pulse–echo ultrasound. Ultrasound waves are pulsed into the body by a transducer. The sonographic image is produced as a result of the reflected echoes that return back to the transducer. (Image reprinted with permission from Brant W. Ultrasound. Philadelphia, PA: Lippincott Williams & Wilkins, 2001:3.)

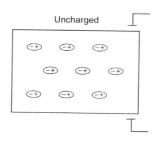
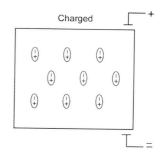

FIGURE 1-11   Piezoelectric crystal. When a voltage is applied across the crystal, the highly polarized molecular dipoles rotate, causing the crystal to thicken and produce ultrasound. Conversely, when ultrasound is received, the mechanical vibration of these structures produces an output voltage. (Image reprinted with permission from Topol EJ, Califf RM, et al. Textbook of Cardiovascular Medicine. 3rd Ed. Philadelphia, PA: Lippincott Williams & Wilkins, 2006.)

a pressure wave (sound) as a result of the vibration of the material. Diagnostic ultrasound uses high-frequency sound waves that are sent into the body by the transducer (transmission), and then the transducer momentarily listens for returning echoes (reflection). The characteristics of the returning echoes are utilized by the ultrasound machine to create an image.

Parameters of Pulsed Sound

Like continuous sound, pulsed sound, or **pulsed wave** (PW) sound, has several specific parameters as well. Parameters of pulsed sound waves include the **pulse repetition frequency**, **pulse repetition period**, **pulse duration**, **duty factor**, and **spatial pulse length** (SPL).

Pulse Repetition Frequency

Remember that frequency is defined as the number of cycles of sound produced in 1 second. The number of pulses of sound produced in 1 second is called the pulse repetition frequency (PRF). Frequency and PRF are not the same. Think of a train made up of five coaches. These represent five pulses. The people on the train represent frequency. Whether there are 2 people (2 Hz) in each coach or 200 (200 Hz), the number of coaches (pulses) stays the same. Therefore, a transducer may produce sound at a frequency of 2 MHz, but it sends out five pulses of this sound every second. Here, the *frequency* is 2 MHz, but the *PRF* is 5 Hz. If it sends out 15 pulses per second, the PRF changes to 15 Hz but the frequency of the sound is still 2 MHz. In diagnostic imaging, the PRF has typical values between 1000 and 10,000 Hz (1 to 10 KHz) (Table 1-21).

The PRF changes whenever the sonographer adjusts the depth control on the ultrasound machine. Recall that when a pulse of sound is emitted, the machine waits for echoes to return before sending out another pulse. If the imaging depth is shallow, the echoes return quickly. If the area of interest is deep, it will take a longer time for the echoes to get back to the transducer. Therefore, the deeper the area of interest, the slower the PRF (Table 1-22). As the imaging depth increases, the PRF decreases, and as the depth decreases, the PRF increases (Figure 1-12).

TABLE 1-21 Pulse repetition frequency.		
Term	**Definition**	**Units**
Pulse repetition frequency	The number of ultrasound pulses emitted in 1 second	Kilohertz (kHz)

TABLE 1-22 Relationship between imaging depth and pulse repetition frequency.
Relationship
↑ Imaging depth ↓ Pulse repetition frequency
↓ Imaging depth ↑ Pulse repetition frequency

FIGURE 1-12 Pulse repetition frequency (PRF). A simple comparison for PRF is the act of bouncing a ball against a wall. If one were to bounce a ball against a wall, standing only 1 ft away from the wall, the rate at which the ball would return would be fairly quick **(A)**. Like ultrasound pulses, you have to wait for the ball to come back before you send it back out again. At 1 ft distance your depth is shallow, and the rate at which you can bounce the ball is very high ($\downarrow$ depth $\uparrow$ PRF). If the distance away from the wall was increased to 15 ft ($\uparrow$ depth), the rate at which you could bounce the ball off of the wall would decrease ($\downarrow$ PRF) **(B)**.

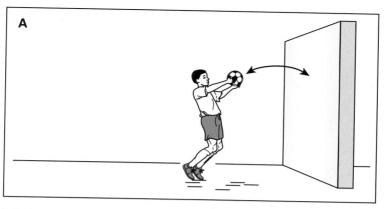

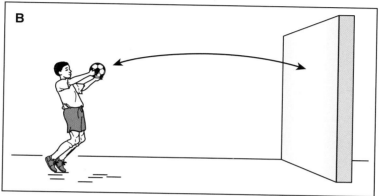

Pulse Repetition Period

Previously, we noted that period is inversely related to frequency. Similarly, the time taken for a pulse to occur is inversely related to the frequency of the pulses. The time taken for a pulse to occur is called the pulse repetition period (PRP) (Figure 1-13). The PRP is the time from the start of one pulse to the start of the next pulse, and therefore, it includes the "on" (or transmit) and "off" (or listening) times (Table 1-23). The relationship that PRP has to PRF is similar to the relationship between period and frequency: when PRP increases, the PRF decreases and vice versa (Table 1-24).

When imaging of superficial structures is performed, the echoes from each pulse return to the transducer quickly, so the time between pulses (PRP) is short. Since the machine is receiving the echoes quickly, it can emit pulses at a faster rate (PRF). Imaging deeper in the body takes a longer time for the echoes to return to the transducer, so the time between pulses, the

FIGURE 1-13 Pulse repetition period. Pulse repetition period is the time of the pulse including the listening time. It is measured from the beginning of one pulse to the beginning of the next pulse.

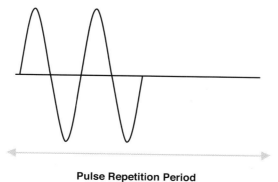

Pulse Repetition Period

TABLE 1-23 Pulsed repetition period.		
Term	**Definition**	**Units**
Pulse repetition period	Time from the beginning of one pulse to the beginning of the next pulse (includes both the "on" and "off" time)	Milliseconds (ms)

TABLE 1-24 Relationship between pulse repetition frequency and pulse repetition period.
Relationship
↑ Pulse repetition frequency ↓ Pulse repetition period
↓ Pulse repetition frequency ↑ Pulse repetition period

TABLE 1-25 Pulse duration.		
Term	**Definition**	**Units**
Pulse duration	Only the active time, or "on" time, that a transducer is pulsing	Microseconds (μs)

PRP, increases. Consequently, the transducer is unable to emit pulses as often so the PRF decreases.

Pulse Duration

While PRP refers to the time from the beginning of one pulse to the beginning of the next, the pulse duration (PD) only relates to the time during which the sound is actually being transmitted, the "on" time (Table 1-25 and Figure 1-14). The duration of the "on" time depends on how many cycles there are in the pulse, and the period of each cycle. The PD is equal to the number of cycles (n) in the pulse multiplied by how long each cycle lasts (period) (Table 1-26).

Pulse Duration

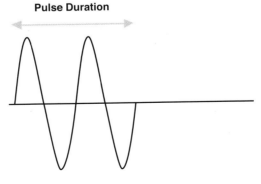

FIGURE 1-14 Pulse duration. Pulse duration is the time of the pulse only during pulse transmission. It is measured from the beginning of one pulse to the end of that pulse.

TABLE 1-26 Formula for pulse duration.
Formula
PD = # of cycles × period
PD = nT

When the crystal in a transducer vibrates or "rings," it produces long pulses with several cycles in each pulse, that is, a long PD. For imaging purposes, a short PD is preferable. To do this, the vibrations of the crystal are damped by a special backing material inside the transducer. The backing or **damping** layer reduces the long "ring" of a vibrating crystal to two or three cycles per pulse. This helps to improve the image by enhancing the **axial resolution**. This is further discussed in Chapter 2. The PD is determined when the transducer is manufactured and cannot be changed by the sonographer.

Duty Factor

The percentage of time that sound is actually being produced is called the duty factor (DF), or duty cycle, and it is equal to PD/PRP (Tables 1-27 and 1-28). If the time between pulses (PRP) is 10.0 μs and the "on" time of the pulse lasts for 5.0 μs, then sound is actually being made 50% of the time from one pulse to another. If the "on" time is reduced to 2.0 μs, then sound is being made only 20% of the time between pulses. If the PRP is short, then the DF will be greater. An ultrasound system with a DF of 100% is CW ultrasound. Pulsed ultrasound will always have a DF less than 100%. In clinical imaging, the DF is 1% or less (Figure 1-15).

Spatial Pulse Length

SPL is defined as the length of a pulse (Table 1-29). The length of the pulse depends on the wavelength of each cycle and the number of cycles in each pulse (Table 1-30). Therefore, SPL equals the number of cycles (n) in the pulse multiplied by the wavelength (λ). If the wavelength increases, the SPL increases and vice versa. If the number of cycles in the pulse increases, then

TABLE 1-27 Duty factor.		
Term	**Definition**	**Units**
Duty factor	The percentage of "on" time only	No unit

TABLE 1-28 Formula for duty factor.
Formula
$\text{Duty factor} = \dfrac{\text{PD}}{\text{PRP}}$

FIGURE 1-15 Duty factor. Comparison between pulse duration, duty factor, and pulse repetition period. Ultrasound energy is usually emitted from the transducer in a series of pulses, each one representing a collection of cycles. Each pulse has a duration and is separated from the next pulse by the dead time. (Image reprinted with permission from Feigenbaum H. Feigenbaum's Echocardiography. 6th Ed. Philadelphia, PA: Lippincott Williams & Wilkins, 2004.)

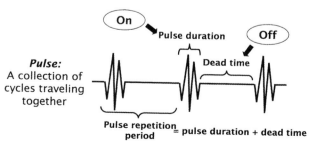

TABLE 1-29 Spatial pulse length.		
Term	Definition	Units
Spatial pulse length	The length of a pulse from beginning to end	Millimeters (mm)

TABLE 1-30 Formula for spatial pulse length.
Formula
SPL = number of cycles × wavelength
SPL = $n\lambda$

the SPL also increases. Either of these would result in a longer lasting pulse or a long PD. SPL, like PD, can be controlled with damping or backing material. Damping reduces the SPL by reducing the number of cycles of each pulse. This damping reduces the PD and SPL and subsequently improves axial resolution. To expand on this concept, remember that the wavelength is inversely related to the frequency of the sound in a given medium. So, higher frequencies have shorter wavelengths and shorter wavelengths result in shorter SPLs. Shorter SPLs mean shorter PDs, which results in better axial resolution and improved overall image quality.

THE SOUND SOURCE AND THE MEDIUM

Parameters of both sound and pulsed sound can be determined by the sound source, the medium through which the sound is traveling, or a combination of both. The sound source simply means the device that is creating the sound. The medium is the tissue through which the sound waves are traveling. Tables 1-31 and 1-32 provide a summary.

TABLE 1-31 Sound wave parameters.		
Determined by Sound Source	Determined by Medium	Determined by Sound Source and Medium
• Period • Frequency • Amplitude, power, and intensity	• Propagation speed • Impedance	• Wavelength

TABLE 1-32 Pulsed sound wave parameters.	
Determined by Sound Source	Determined by Sound Source and Medium
• Pulse duration • Duty factor • Pulse repetition period • Pulse repetition frequency	• Spatial pulse length

INTERACTIONS OF SOUND WITH TISSUE

Attenuation and Absorption

Attenuation is a decrease in the amplitude, power, and intensity of the sound beam as sound travels through tissue. There are three mechanisms of attenuation: **absorption**, reflection, and **scattering**. When evaluating two intensities, such as powers or amplitudes, the units of **decibels (dB)** are used. Decibels imply that one thing is being compared to another, such as the initial intensity and the end intensity. If an intensity or power doubles, it has changed by 3 dB. Similarly, if an intensity or power decreases by half, it has changed by −3 dB. Table 1-33 provides a summary of dB changes.

Absorption, the conversion of sound energy to heat, is the greatest contributor to attenuation in tissue. It is also a potential source of thermal bioeffects, as will be discussed in further detail in Chapter 6. The amount of attenuation that occurs as sound travels is related to the frequency of the beam. It is important to remember that high-frequency transducers do not penetrate as well as lower-frequency transducers.

The **attenuation coefficient** (in dB/cm) is the rate at which sound is attenuated per unit depth. It is equal to one half of the frequency ($f/2$) in soft tissue. The **total attenuation** is the total amount of sound (in dB) that has been attenuated at a given depth. To determine the total attenuation, one needs to know the rate and the **path length**.

The purpose of a toll road as a taxation mechanism can be used to demonstrate the total attenuation of the sound beam. For example, if someone wanted to drive on the Garden State Parkway in New Jersey from Asbury Park to Cape May, they would have to pay certain tolls. If a toll of $1.00 was applied to every mile, the toll, or rate, is $1.00 per mile, and it does not change with distance. (This is analogous to the attenuation coefficient, which is the toll sound pays for every centimeter of depth.) If someone traveled 140 miles from Asbury Park to Cape May, the total toll paid (similar to the total attenuation) is $140.

If the rate of attenuation is known (attenuation coefficient in dB/cm, which is equal to $f/2$ in soft tissue) and the path length (in cm) is known as well, the total attenuation (in dB) can be calculated (Table 1-34). The average rate of attenuation in soft tissue is 0.7 dB/cm/MHz.

Specular and Nonspecular Reflectors

An interface is the dividing line between two different media. At the interface, sound may be absorbed, reflected, scattered, transmitted, or refracted.

TABLE 1-33 Decibel chart for intensity/power.

Increasing Intensity/Power		Decreasing Intensity/Power	
0 dB	No change	−0 dB	No change
3 dB	Double	−3 dB	One half
6 dB	Quadruple	−6 dB	One fourth
10 dB	10 times	−10 dB	One tenth
20 dB	100 times	−20 dB	One hundredth

TABLE 1-34 Formula for attenuation coefficient.	
Formula	**Example**
Total attenuation = Attenuation coefficient (Ac) × path length (L) $$TA = \frac{f}{2} \times L$$	If a 10-MHz sound travels through soft tissue, how much total attenuation has occurred at a depth of 5 cm? Attenuation coefficient = f/2 = 10 MHz/2 = 5 dB/cm Total attenuation = f/2 × L = 5 dB/cm × 5 cm = 25 dB

FIGURE 1-16 Reflection and scattering. The interaction between an ultrasound wave and its target depends on several factors. A specular reflection occurs when ultrasound encounters a target that is large relative to the transmitted wavelength. The amount of ultrasound energy that is reflected to the transducer by a specular target depends on the angle and the impedance of the tissue. Targets that are small relative to the transmitted wavelength produce a scattering of ultrasound energy, resulting in a small portion of energy being returned to the transducer. This type of interaction results in "speckle" that produces the texture within tissues. (Image reprinted with permission from Feigenbaum H. Feigenbaum's Echocardiography. 6th Ed. Philadelphia, PA: Lippincott Williams & Wilkins, 2004.)

Reflectors in the medium are often referred to as being either specular or nonspecular reflectors.

Specular reflections occur when the sound impinges upon a large, smooth reflector at a 90° angle. (Specular is Latin for "mirror.") A large specular reflector is one in which the size of the reflector is larger than the wavelength of the incident beam (Figure 1-16). Examples of specular reflectors are the diaphragm, the capsules of organs, and the wall of the aorta (Table 1-35). Specular reflectors are highly angle dependent. That is, if the sound strikes a reflector at an oblique angle, the reflection will not return to the transducer. Therefore, the best 2D images come from striking a reflector perpendicular to the interface.

Nonspecular reflectors are ones in which their size is smaller than the wavelength of the incident beam. The parenchyma of an organ is an example of nonspecular reflectors. Nonspecular reflectors scatter sound in many different directions. Some of this sound, termed **backscatter**, makes it back to the transducer and produces an image on the display. The intensity of backscatter is much lower than the intensity from specular reflectors, although nonspecular reflectors are not angle dependent as are the

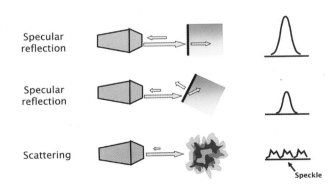

TABLE 1-35 Specular versus nonspecular reflectors.	
Specular Reflectors	**Nonspecular Reflectors**
Smooth surface	Rough surface
Border is larger than incident wavelength	Border is smaller than incident wavelength
Angle dependent	Not angle dependent

specular reflectors. Scatter permits the imaging of the parenchyma, while specular reflectors are the boundaries. When sound strikes a number of scatterers, the scatter waves interact with each other (constructively and destructively) and send the result of these interactions back to the transducer. This interference pattern is termed **acoustic speckle** and appears as "parenchyma" on the screen. In other words, when imaging a liver, the tiny dots on the screen that represent liver tissue do not actually represent the liver cells themselves but are the result of all of the scattering reflectors interfering with each other (Figure 1-17). Manufacturers have employed "speckle reduction" algorithms to try to smooth out the appearance of speckle in the image and create a smoother-appearing image (Figure 1-18).

With higher-frequency transducers, there is a higher intensity of scatter. For this reason, higher-frequency transducers are limited to shallower depths. If the energy of the beam is scattered, there is a reduction in the amount of sound that remains to be transmitted through the tissue. Very small reflectors, like red blood cells, are termed **Rayleigh scatterers**. Rayleigh scatterers scatter sound equally in all directions (omnidirectional). With Rayleigh scatterers, as the frequency increases, the intensity of scatter increases proportional to the fourth power of the frequency.

FIGURE 1-17 Acoustic speckle. Acoustic speckle is formed as a result of the interference pattern from multiple interfering scatterers. This gives parenchyma its characteristic look on a sonogram. (Images courtesy of Dr. Asbjorn Stoylen. Available at: http://folk.ntnu. no/stoylen/strainrate/ Ultrasound/.)

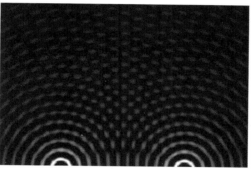
Interference pattern of two reflectors

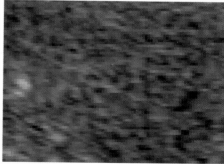
Parenchyma, magnified

FIGURE 1-18 Speckle reduction. Speckle reduction algorithms to try to smooth out the appearance of speckle in the image **(A)** and create a smoother-appearing image **(B)**. (Image used with permission from GE Healthcare.)

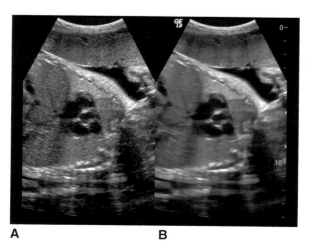

A   B

More about Reflection

A reflection is formed when two criteria are met: there is **normal incidence** and the two media have different impedances. Synonyms for normal incidence include orthogonal, perpendicular, and 90°. If there is no change in impedance, then there is no reflection, and all of the sound is transmitted through the tissue. Sound that is transmitted travels through the tissue in the same direction as it was transmitted, and reflected sound returns to the source. That is to say, the angle of reflection equals the angle of incidence.

Oblique incidence is complex, and reflection/transmission of sound cannot be predicted. Any sound that is reflected with an oblique angle of incidence does not return to the transducer. However, as with normal incidence, the angle of reflection equals the angle of incidence ($\theta_r = \theta_i$). Two types of oblique angles are acute (<90°) and obtuse (>90°).

The intensity of sound reflected at an interface is dependent upon the intensity of the transmitted sound and the difference in impedances between the two media. The bigger the impedance mismatch, the stronger the reflection. The percentage of sound transmitted at an interface, or **intensity transmission coefficient** (ITC) is equal to 1 minus the percentage of sound reflected at an interface, or **intensity reflection coefficient** (IRC) (Table 1-36). The IRC plus the ITC must equal 100%. If the impedances of the media are the same, then there is no reflection, and the ITC = 100%. Table 1-37 provides the equation used to calculate percentage or intensity of reflected sound.

Refraction

Refraction is a redirection of the transmitted sound beam. Refraction should not be confused with reflection (Table 1-38). With normal incidence, the transmitted beam angle is equal to the incident angle. When sound strikes an interface with an oblique angle of incidence, the transmitted beam angle will equal the incident angle only if the propagation speeds are identical. If there is oblique incidence and a propagation speed mismatch, the transmitted angle will be different from the incident angle. In theory, if the propagation speed of medium 2 is *less than* the propagation speed of

T A B L E 1 - 3 6 Intensity transmission coefficient.	
Formula	**Example**
ITC = 1 − IRC	Sound travels through an interface at normal incidence and 40% of the sound is reflected back to the transducer. How much sound was transmitted at the interface? ITC = 1 − 40% = 60%

T A B L E 1 - 3 7   Intensity reflection coefficient.
Formula
$$IRC = \frac{I_r}{I_i} = \left[\frac{Z_2 - Z_1}{Z_2 + Z_1} \right]^2$$

TABLE 1-38 Reflection versus refraction.	
Reflection	**Refraction**
• Normal (perpendicular) incidence • Impedance mismatch • Percentage or intensity of sound reflected and transmitted at an interface	• Oblique incidence • Propagation speed mismatch • Angle of transmitted sound

FIGURE 1-19 Refraction. If the propagation speed of medium 2 is *less than* the propagation speed of medium 1, then the angle of transmission will be *less than* the angle of incidence **(A)**. Likewise, if the propagation speed of medium 2 is *greater than* the propagation speed of medium 1, then the angle of transmission will be *greater than* the angle of incidence **(B)**. (Image used with permission from GE Healthcare.)

A $\quad \theta_t < \theta_i \text{ if } C_2 < C_1$

B $\quad \theta_t > \theta_i \text{ if } C_2 > C_1$

TABLE 1-39 Snell's law.
Formula
$\sin \theta_t = \sin \theta_i \dfrac{C_2}{C_1}$

medium 1, then the angle of transmission will be *less than* the angle of incidence. Likewise, if the propagation speed of medium 2 is *greater than* the propagation speed of medium 1, then the angle of transmission will be *greater than* the angle of incidence (Figure 1-19). **Snell's law** describes the angle of transmission at an interface based on the angle of incidence and the propagation speeds of the two media (Table 1-39).

MORE ABOUT INTENSITY

With PW sound operation, the intensity of the beam varies with space and time. Simply acknowledging that the intensity of an ultrasound beam is 100 mW/cm^2 is not always enough information. Many times, it must be specified as to *where* and *when* the sound beam was measured. The spatial intensities, spatial average (SA), and spatial peak (SP), refer to *where* the beam was measured. The SP intensity is measured at the center of the beam. Often, a flashlight analogy is utilized. If one were to look at the center of the flashlight, they would notice that the center of the flashlight yields the brightest light, or most intense light. This is much how the ultrasound beam is shaped. That is, the strongest intensity is in the center of the beam and gradually reduces as the beam spreads out. The SA intensity is the average intensity across the face of the entire beam. The beam uniformity ratio (BUR), also referred to as the SP/SA factor or beam uniformity coefficient (BUC), is the ratio of the center intensity to the average spatial intensity (Table 1-40).

The temporal intensities depict when the beam was measured. The temporal peak (TP) is the intensity measured at the highest intensity, or peak, of the pulse and is therefore the highest of all the temporal intensities. The

TABLE 1-40 Beam uniformity ratio.
Formula
$$BUR = \frac{SP}{SA}$$

The beam uniformity ratio (BUR) is derived from dividing the spatial peak (SP) by the spatial average (SA).

temporal average (TA) is the average of all the intensities during both transmission and the listening period. It is important to note that when the transducer is waiting for the pulse to come back, the intensity is zero because sound is only produced during transmission phase. Because the beam is only transmitting less than 1% of the time in PW operation, the TA is the lowest of all the temporal intensities. This means that 99% of the time, the intensity is zero. The pulse average (PA) is measured only during beam transmission. The formula for TA is provided in Table 1-41. The TA is equal to the PA times the DF. With CW operation, where the DF is equal to 1, the TA is equal to the PA because there is no listening time.

When grouped together, the spatial and temporal intensities provide a specific explanation for the measurement of the intensity of the sound beam in both space and time. For example, the SATA intensity signifies that the beam was measured using the SA and TA intensities. Table 1-42 lists the order of intensities from lowest to highest. It is most important to note that SATA is the lowest of the intensities, SPTP is the highest, and the SPTA intensity is used when describing thermal bioeffects. Intensity, and its association with bioeffects, will be discussed further in Chapter 6 of this book.

The **hydrophone**, or microprobe, is a device used to measure output intensity of the transducer (Figure 1-20). It can be a needle-type device or a broad, disk-shaped device. Both types of hydrophones consist of a transducer that is placed into the path of the beam to measure PRP, PD, and period. From these measurements, other parameters, such as frequency, wavelength, SPL, PRF, and DF, can be derived. The hydrophone is also used to determine pressure amplitude and intensities, which are important for patient safety.

TABLE 1-41 Temporal average formula
Formula
$$TA = PA \times DF$$

The temporal average (TA) is equal to the pulse average (PA) multiplied by the duty factor (DF).

TABLE 1-42 The list of intensities from lowest (SATA) to highest (SPTP).
Intensities from Lowest to Highest
SATA > SPTA > SAPA > SPPA > SATP > SPTP

FIGURE 1-20 Intensities. **A.** Pressure amplitude variations are measured with a hydrophone and include peak compression and rarefaction variations with time. **B.** Temporal intensity variations of pulsed ultrasound vary widely, from temporal peak and temporal average values; pulse average intensity represents the average intensity measured over the pulse duration. **C.** Spatial intensity variations of pulsed ultrasound are described by the spatial peak value and the spatial average value, measured over the ultrasound beam.

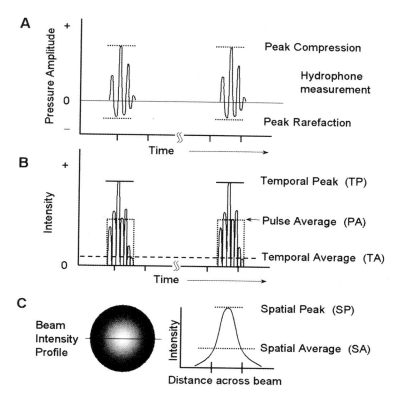

REVIEW QUESTIONS

1. Which of the following is described as the ability of an object to resist compression and relates to the hardness of a medium?
   a. Stiffness
   b. Density
   c. Pressure
   d. Inertia

2. An increase in pulse repetition frequency would lead to:
   a. An increase in duty factor
   b. An increase in pulse duration
   c. An increase in the number of cycles
   d. A decrease in resolution

3. Which of the following would have the highest propagation speed?
   a. Air
   b. Bone
   c. Soft tissue
   d. Water

4. Which of the following would have the lowest propagation speed?
   a. Water
   b. Soft tissue
   c. Bone
   d. Lung tissue

5. As imaging depth increases, the pulse repetition frequency must:
   a. Not change
   b. Increase
   c. Decrease
   d. Pulse repetition frequency does not relate to imaging depth

6. Which of the following describes the amount of refraction that occurs at an interface?
   a. Bernoulli's law
   b. Poiseuille's law
   c. Law of reflection
   d. Snell's law

7. Pressure is typically expressed in:
   a. Frequency
   b. Pascals
   c. Decibels
   d. Kilograms per centimeter cubed

8. The typical range of frequency for diagnostic ultrasound imaging is:
   a. 20 to 20,000 Hz
   b. 1 to 20 MHz
   c. 10 to 20 MHz
   d. 12 to 100 MHz

9. The attenuation coefficient in soft tissue is equal to:
   a. One half of the operating frequency
   b. Double the operating frequency
   c. Frequency times path length
   d. The total decibels

10. Micro denotes:
    a. Millionth
    b. Hundredth
    c. Million
    d. Billionth

11. Which of the following is described as the distance over which one cycle occurs?
    a. Pulse duration
    b. Duty factor
    c. Period
    d. Wavelength

12. All of the following are true of stiffness except:
    a. It is defined as the ability of an object to resist compression
    b. Stiffness and propagation speed are indirectly associated
    c. Increasing stiffness increases propagation speed
    d. Stiffness may also be referred to as elasticity

13. Areas of high pressure and density are referred to as:
    a. Compressions
    b. Rarefactions
    c. Condensations
    d. Rarefractions

14. Spatial pulse length can be calculated by:
    a. Multiplying the number of cycles times the frequency
    b. Dividing the period by the frequency
    c. Multiplying the number of cycles times the wavelength
    d. Dividing the number of cycles by the wavelength

15. Density is typically measured in:
    a. Kilograms per centimeter cubed
    b. Millimeters

c. Watts per centimeter squared
d. Pascals

16. As a sound wave travels through the human body, the intensity of the sound wave decreases as a result of:
a. Attenuation
b. Absorption
c. Scattering
d. All of the above

17. What is the total amount of attenuation that occurs if a 6.0-MHz sound beam travels through 4 cm of soft tissue?
a. 24 dB
b. 12 dB
c. 6 dB
d. None of the above

18. As imaging depth increases, pulse repetition period:
a. Remains constant
b. Increases
c. Decreases
d. Doubles

19. If pulse repetition frequency increases, then the duty factor:
a. Remains constant
b. Increases
c. Decreases
d. Doubles

20. The *percentage* of time that the ultrasound system is producing pulses of ultrasound describes the:
a. Pulse repetition period
b. Pulse duration
c. Duty factor
d. Pulse repetition frequency

21. Density and propagation speed are:
a. Inversely related
b. Directly related
c. Directly proportional
d. Unrelated

22. All of the following are true of power except:
a. As amplitude increases, power remains the same
b. Power is proportional to amplitude squared
c. Intensity is proportional to power
d. Power is measured in milliwatts

23. All of the following are true of wavelength except:
a. It is determined by both the medium and the sound source
b. It is equal to the period divided by the frequency
c. It is inversely related to frequency
d. It is directly related to period

24. Which of the following is determined by the sound source and medium?
a. Propagation speed
b. Frequency

c. Period
d. Wavelength

25. Which of the following is defined as the number of ultrasound pulses emitted in 1 second?
a. Pulse repetition period
b. Duty factor
c. Pulse repetition frequency
d. Spatial pulse length

26. Which of the following is defined as only the active time?
a. Duty factor
b. Pulse repetition frequency
c. Period
d. Pulse duration

27. The inertia of the medium describes its:
a. Attenuation characteristics
b. Stiffness
c. Density
d. Elasticity

28. Which of the following is determined by the sound source only?
a. Frequency
b. Wavelength
c. Spatial pulse length
d. Propagation speed

29. The prefix "centi" denotes:
a. Thousandths
b. Hundredths
c. Millions
d. Hundreds

30. If the angle of incidence is 40°, what is the angle of transmission at the interface if medium 1 has a propagation speed of 1320 m/s and medium 2 has a propagation speed of 1700 m/s?
a. <40°
b. >40°
c. 40°
d. Cannot tell the angle of transmission

31. The change in the direction of the original sound wave that occurs when sound interacts with two different tissue types that have a different propagation speed is referred to as:
a. Wavelength
b. Scattering
c. Refraction
d. Absorption

32. Which of the following is an appropriate unit of measurement for propagation speed?
a. millimeters per microsecond (mm/μs)
b. watts per centimeter squared (W/cm^2)
c. microseconds (μs)
d. kilohertz (kHz)

33. The major component of attenuation is:
    a. Scatter
    b. Absorption
    c. Transmission
    d. Refraction

34. In clinical imaging, the wavelength measures between:
    a. 1 and 10 Hz
    b. 1540 and 2000 m/s
    c. 0 and 1
    d. 0.1 to 0.8 mm

35. The duty factor for continuous wave ultrasound is:
    a. <99%
    b. 100%
    c. >20,000 Hz
    d. 8 Pa

36. All of the following relate to the strength of the sound wave except:
    a. Amplitude
    b. Wavelength
    c. Intensity
    d. Power

37. What is the change in intensity if the power decreases by half?
    a. Intensity doubles
    b. Intensity is halved
    c. Intensity is one fourth
    d. Intensity does not change

38. Damping of the sound beam:
    a. Reduces the spatial pulse length
    b. Increases the spatial pulse length
    c. Increases the pulse duration
    d. Has no impact on spatial pulse length or pulse duration

39. What is defined as the ability of the ultrasound system to image structures that are positioned parallel to the sound beam as separate structures?
    a. Transverse resolution
    b. Parallel resolution
    c. Axial resolution
    d. Coronal resolution

40. What is defined as the beginning of one pulse to the beginning of the next pulse, and therefore includes both the "on" and "off" time?
    a. Pulse repetition period
    b. Pulse duration
    c. Duty factor
    d. Pulse repetition frequency

41. What is pressure measured in?
    a. feet, inches, centimeters, or miles
    b. pascals or pounds per square inch
    c. kilograms per centimeter cubed
    d. hertz, kilohertz, or megahertz

42. What is essentially equal to the power of a wave divided by the area over which the power is distributed?
    a. Amplitude
    b. Power
    c. Intensity
    d. Absorption

43. Transducers have material within them that, when electronically stimulated, produces ultrasound waves. This is most likely some form of:
    a. Copperhirm titonize
    b. Zinconian sulfate
    c. Lead zirconate titanate
    d. Barium

44. What is the change in power if the amplitude triples?
    a. It doubles
    b. It triples
    c. It quadruples
    d. It increases nine times

45. The portion of the sound beam where the molecules are pulled apart describes an area of:
    a. Compression
    b. Rarefaction
    c. Refraction
    d. Amplitude

46. If only the density of a medium is increased, then the:
    a. Propagation speed will increase
    b. Propagation speed will decrease
    c. Propagation speed will stay the same
    d. None of the above

47. Sound is technically a:
    a. Transverse and longitudinal wave
    b. Mechanical and transverse wave
    c. Nonmechanical and pressure wave
    d. Mechanical and longitudinal wave

48. The maximum value or minimum value of an acoustic variable minus the equilibrium value of that variable describes the:
    a. Power
    b. Intensity
    c. Duty factor
    d. Amplitude

49. Which of the following would be considered ultrasonic?
    a. 10 Hz
    b. 12.5 Hz
    c. 1 MHz
    d. 200 Hz

50. Which of the following is considered the speed of sound in soft tissue?
    a. 660 m/s
    b. 330 m/s
    c. 1480 m/s
    d. 1540 m/s

SUGGESTED READINGS

Brant W. The Core Curriculum: Ultrasound. Philadelphia, PA: Lippincott Williams & Wilkins, 2001.

Case T. A Primer in Ultrasound and Vascular Physics. Philadelphia, PA: Lippincott Williams & Wilkins, 2007.

Edelman SK. Understanding Ultrasound Physics. 3rd Ed. Woodlands, TX: ESP Inc., 2005.

Rosen J. Encyclopedia of Physics. New York, NY: Facts on File Inc., 2004.

Kremkau FW. Diagnostic Ultrasound: Principles and Instruments. 7th Ed. St. Louis, MO: Saunders, 2006.

Ultrasound Transducers

INTRODUCTION

This chapter will describe the way in which sound is produced by the transducer, including construction of the transducer, image resolution, and care and maintenance of the transducer.

KEY TERMS

aperture—the diameter of the piezoelectric element(s) producing the beam

array—the transducer with multiple active elements

automatic scanning—same as real-time ultrasound

axial resolution—the ability to accurately identify reflectors that are arranged parallel to the ultrasound beam

backing material—the damping material of the transducer assembly, which reduces the number of cycles produced in a pulse

bandwidth—the range of frequencies present within the beam

constructive interference—occurs when in-phase waves meet; the amplitudes of the two waves are added to form one large wave

contrast resolution—the ability to differentiate one shade of gray from another

crystal—a synonym for the active element of the transducer, the piezoelectric part of the transducer assembly that produces sound

Curie point—the temperature at which an ultrasound transducer will gain its piezoelectric properties, and also the temperature at which a transducer will lose the ability to produce sound if heated again above this temperature

curved sequenced array—the transducer commonly referred to as curvilinear or convex probe

damping—the process of reducing the number of cycles of each pulse in order to improve axial resolution

damping material—same as backing material, the part of transducer assembly that reduces the number of cycles produced in a pulse

depth ambiguity—the inability to determine the depth of the reflector if the pulses are sent out too fast for them to be timed

destructive interference—occurs when out-of-phase waves meet; the amplitude of the resultant wave is smaller than either of the original waves

diffraction—spreading of the beam that occurs after the focal zone

divergence—spreading of the beam that occurs in the far zone

element—the piezoelectric part of the transducer assembly that produces sound

elevational plane—*see* key term slice-thickness plane

elevational resolution—the resolution in the third dimension of the beam: the slice-thickness plane

far zone—the diverging part of the beam distal to the focal point

focal point—the area of the beam with the smallest beam diameter

footprint—the portion of the transducer that is in contact with the patient's skin

frame—one complete ultrasound image

frame rate—the number of frames per second

Fraunhofer zone—*see* key term far zone

frequency—the number of cycles per second

Fresnel zone—*see* key term near zone

Huygen's principle—states that waves are the result of the interference of many wavelets produced at the face of the transducer

in-phase—waves whose peaks and troughs overlap

lateral resolution—the ability to accurately identify reflectors that are arranged perpendicular to the ultrasound beam

lead zirconate titanate—abbreviated as PZT, this is the man-made ceramic of which many transducer elements are made

linear phased array—the transducer that uses phasing, or small time differences, to steer and focus the beam

linear sequenced array—the transducer commonly referred to as a "linear probe"

matching layer—the component of the transducer that is used to step down the impedance from that of the element to that of the patient's skin

mechanical scanheads—transducers with a motor for steering the beam

near zone—the part of the beam between the element and the focal point

near zone length—the length of the region from the transducer face to the focal point

out-of-phase—waves that are 180° opposite each other; the peak of one wave overlaps the trough of the other and vice versa

phasing—the method of focusing and/or steering the beam by applying electrical impulses to the piezoelectric elements with small time differences between shocks

piezoelectric—the ability to convert pressure into electricity and electricity into pressure

quality factor (Q-factor)—a measure of beam purity; the operating frequency of the transducer divided by the bandwidth

real-time—live ultrasound, also known as "automatic scanning"

scan lines—created when one or more pulses of sound return from the tissue containing information related to the depth and amplitude of the reflectors

section-thickness plane—*see* slice-thickness plane

sensitivity—the ability of a system to display low-level or weak echoes

shock excitation—applying electrical energy to the piezoelectric element causes it to resonate

slice-thickness plane—the third dimension of the beam

spatial pulse length—the length of the pulse

spatial resolution—refers to axial, lateral, contrast, and elevational resolution

temporal resolution—also known as frame rate, ability to display moving structures in real time

transducer—any device that converts one form of energy into another. May also refer to the part of the ultrasound machine that produces sound

tungsten—component of the backing material

wavefront—the leading edge of a wave, formed as a result of Huygen's principle, which is perpendicular to the direction of the propagating wave

wavelet—a small wave created as a result of Huygen's principle

THE PIEZOELECTRIC ELEMENT AND THE PRODUCTION OF SOUND

The Piezoelectric Element

A **piezoelectric** material, as mentioned in Chapter 1, is an element that generates electricity when pressure is applied to it and that changes shape when electricity is applied to it. The piezoelectric material is the material that produces diagnostic ultrasound. Piezoelectric materials may be naturally occurring, such as quartz and tourmaline, or man-made. The piezoelectric material that is commonly used in current ultrasound transducers is a man-made ceramic called **lead zirconate titanate** (PZT). The PZT is the actual transducer inside the scanhead. It may also be referred to as the **crystal**, the **element**, or simply, the **transducer**.

The piezoelectric material must undergo a process to obtain its piezoelectric properties. First, the PZT is placed into an oven that is used to heat the material to the **Curie point**. The Curie point is the temperature at which the material will obtain piezoelectric properties. While being heated, the PZT is placed into a magnetic field. This causes magnetically charged molecules, called dipoles, that are located within the material, to align themselves in relation to the magnetic field. Once the material is cooled, it is functional as a piezoelectric element. Unfortunately, once a ceramic is taken to its Curie point, it must never return to that temperature again or the material will lose its piezoelectric properties forever. For this reason, ultrasound transducers are never heat sterilized. When necessary, transducers must be cold sterilized using either a glutaraldehyde solution, such as Cidex or Metricide, or a non–glutaraldehyde-based solution, such as *ortho*-phthalaldehyde (Figure 2-1). Cold-sterilizing solutions can be dangerous if they get on the skin or are inhaled. Personal protective equipment must be worn while handling these solutions. Sonographers should be familiar with the appropriate material safety data sheets for these solutions.

Production of Sound

One or more piezoelectric elements are attached to an electric wire in the transducer. Applying electricity to the element causes it to resonate, or alternatively expand and contract. This is called **shock excitation**. The **frequency**, or rate at which the material resonates is related to two factors: the thickness of the piezoelectric element and the propagation speed of the element itself

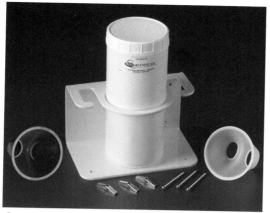
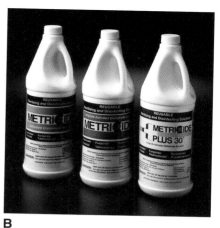

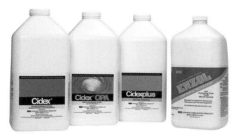

FIGURE 2-1 Ultrasound transducers are placed in a container **(A)** and must be cold sterilized using various chemicals **(B,C)**.
B and C are photos of cold-sterilization fluids. (Photos courtesy of CIVCO Medical Solutions.)

(Table 2-1). In pulsed-wave operation, the thickness of the element is the primary determinant of the resonating frequency of the transducer. A thicker element will produce a lower frequency, whereas a thinner element will produce a higher frequency (Figure 2-2). The operator cannot change the resonating frequency of a piezoelectric element.

The resonating element produces a pressure wave. This wave consists of alternating waves of high pressure and low pressure, or compressions and rarefactions, respectively. The resonating frequency, also known as the center or operating frequency, of a medical diagnostic ultrasound transducer is typically between 2 and 15 MHz. This expanding and contracting of the element produces a propagating ultrasound wave that travels into the human body.

Many ultrasound transducers use pulsed sound. Piezoelectric elements can both send and receive ultrasound but not at the same time. That is, a single element can emit sound, but it must wait for that sound to return before it can send out the next pulse. The machine must time how long it takes for a pulse of sound to reach the reflector in order to appropriately display

T A B L E **2 - 1** Formula for the frequency of the transducer for pulsed-wave operation. The operating frequency (F_o) is equal to the propagation speed (c) of the element divided by the thickness of the element multiplied by 2.
Formula
$F_o = c/2 \times$ thickness

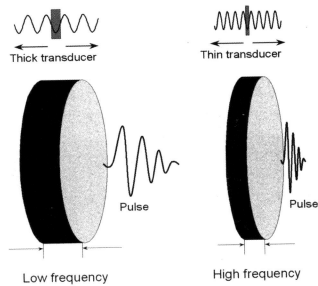

f_o is determined by the transducer thickness equal to ½ λ

Thick transducer

Thin transducer

Pulse

Pulse

Low frequency

High frequency

FIGURE 2-2   Transducer elements. The thicker the element, the lower the frequency, and the thinner the element, the higher the frequency. (Image reprinted with permission from Bushberg J. The Essential Physics of Medical Imaging. 2nd Ed. Philadelphia, PA: Lippincott Williams & Wilkins, 2002:486.)

anatomy on the monitor. If the transducer sends out a pulse before it receives the last one, it is unable to recognize where the echo originated, and therefore, cannot display it correctly on the monitor. This is referred to as **depth ambiguity**.

Huygen's Principle

As stated in Chapter 1, sound travels as a wave. These waves may interact with each other. Subsequently, these waves may be described further as **in-phase** or **out-of-phase**. In-phase waves are waves that, when stacked, have matching peaks and troughs (Figure 2-3). When in-phase waves meet, they undergo **constructive interference**, that is, they become one big wave. Out-of-phase waves, when overlapped, are 180 degrees opposite each other (Figure 2-4). When out-of-phase waves meet, they undergo **destructive interference**. With destructive interference, the resultant wave is smaller. Also, if the out-of-phase waves have identical amplitudes, they can even completely cancel each other out.

The surface of the transducer is made up of many, tiny point sources of sound. Each tiny point on the transducer produces a **wavelet**. All of the wavelets that are created undergo either constructive or destructive

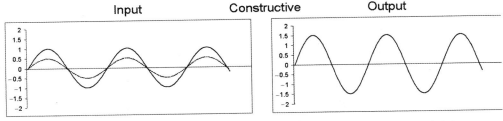

Input   Constructive   Output

FIGURE 2-3   Demonstration of two in-phase waves. The amplitudes of the two waves are added together, which results in one large wave. (Image reprinted with permission from Bushberg J. The Essential Physics of Medical Imaging. 2nd Ed. Philadelphia, PA: Lippincott Williams & Wilkins, 2002:474.)

Destructive

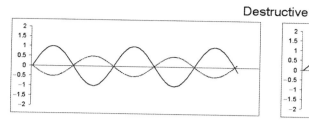 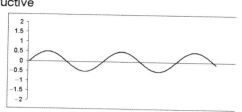

FIGURE 2-4 Demonstration of two out-of-phase waves. With nonidentical waves, as demonstrated in this image, the resultant wave has a smaller amplitude than the two initial waves. With identical waves, they cancel each other out. (Image reprinted with permission from Bushberg J. The Essential Physics of Medical Imaging. 2nd Ed. Philadelphia, PA: Lippincott Williams & Wilkins, 2002:474.)

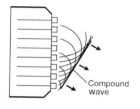

FIGURE 2-5 Huygen's principle. The beam starts out as small wavelets at the face of the transducer. The interference of the wavelets produces a propagation sound beam. The direction in which the beam travels is perpendicular to the wavefront. (Image reprinted with permission from Topol EJ, Califf RM. Textbook of Cardiovascular Medicine. 3rd Ed. Philadelphia, PA: Lippincott Williams & Wilkins, 2006.)

interference. The end result is a propagating sound wave whose direction of travel is perpendicular to the **wavefront**, which is the line tangential to all the wavelets (Figure 2-5). This is referred to as **Huygen's principle**.

CONSTRUCTION OF THE TRANSDUCER

The various components of the transducer can be seen in Figure 2-6 and are further discussed in detail in the following sections and described in Table 2-2.

Transducer Housing and the Wire

Diagnostic ultrasound instruments use electricity to generate an image. The ultrasound machine produces between 10 and 500 V in order to drive the piezoelectric elements. If a crack occurs in the transducer housing, there is a potential risk for electrical shock to either the practitioner or the patient. Consequently, the ultrasound transducer is insulated not only to protect the image from outside electrical interference but also to protect both the user and the patient.

An electrical connection to the ultrasound machine is achieved via a wire (Figure 2-7). Modern scanheads often contain more than a hundred individual transducer elements, each of which is supplied with electrical energy via a wire. This wire also transmits the received echo amplitude information to the machine for processing. A flexible sheathed connector is located at the point at which the wire connects to the transducer. The importance of the connector is to allow flexibility of the cord and prevent damage to the wire where it connects to the transducer.

FIGURE 2-6 Construction of the transducer. (Image reprinted with permission from Feigenbaum H. Feigenbaum's Echocardiography. 6th Ed. Philadelphia, PA: Lippincott Williams & Wilkins, 2004.)

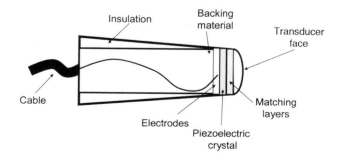

TABLE 2-2 Summary of the transducer assembly.	
Transducer Part	**Purpose**
Backing material	Shortens the length of the pulse by decreasing the number of cycles in the pulse
Crystal	Material that produces diagnostic ultrasound. Composed of piezoelectric material, most commonly lead zirconate titanate. Converts electrical energy into acoustic energy during transmission and acoustic energy into electrical energy during reception
Housing	Provides insulation and protection from electrical shock
Matching layer	Used to step down the impedance from that of the element to that of the patient's skin
Wire	Used to transfer electrical signals to and from the transducer

Matching Layer

It is important to remember that the bigger the impedance mismatch, the stronger the reflection. The more sound that is reflected off of the skin, the less sound there is to be transmitted into the tissue. The impedance of the piezoelectric element is significantly different from that of the patient's skin. If no action were taken, this large mismatch would prevent almost all of the sound from entering the patient. Actually, 80% of the sound would be reflected and only 20% would be transmitted into the patient. Therefore, the transducer is equipped with a **matching layer** that lies between the piezoelectric element and the patient's skin. Although often referred to as if it were a single layer, the matching layer is actually composed of multiple layers (Figure 2-8). The purpose of the layers is to step down the impedance from that of the element to that of the patient's skin. The matching layer improves the efficiency of transmitting sound into the patient by decreasing this impedance mismatch. An additional matching layer, employed by the sonographer, is the coupling medium, or gel. In addition to removing air between the transducer and the patient, gel is specially formulated to have an impedance value between that of the matching layer and the patient's skin to further enhance the transmission of sound.

FIGURE 2-7 The wires of the transducer. Note that each element is connected by a wire. (Image reprinted with permission from Feigenbaum H. Feigenbaum's Echocardiography. 6th Ed. Philadelphia, PA: Lippincott Williams & Wilkins, 2004.)

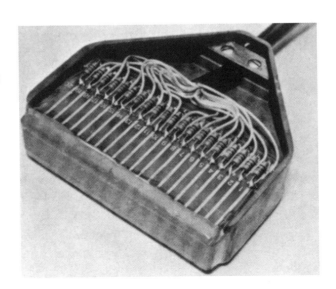

FIGURE 2-8 Enlarged diagram of the construction of the transducer. This diagram depicts the multiple layers that create the matching layer. (Image reprinted with permission from Sanders R. Clinical Sonography: A Practical Guide. 4th Ed. Philadelphia, PA: Lippincott Williams & Wilkins, 2007:9.)

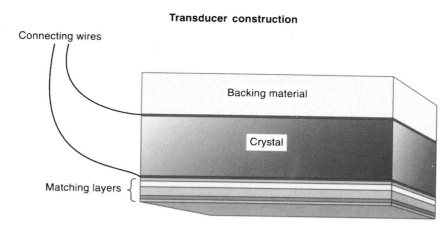

Transducer construction

Connecting wires

Backing material

Crystal

Matching layers

T A B L E 2 - 3 Advantages of damping.
Advantages of Damping
Decreases the number of cycles in a pulse
Decreases spatial pulse length
Increases axial resolution

Backing Material and Damping

The backing material, as the name implies, sits on the back of the transducer, behind the elements (Figure 2-8). The purpose of the **backing material**, or **damping material**, is to provide **damping** of the piezoelectric element. The damping material serves to shorten the length of the pulse by decreasing the number of cycles in the pulse. This material is composed of an epoxy resin loaded with **tungsten**.

There are several advantages of damping (Table 2-3). The element can be compared to a bell. When a bell is struck, it will keep ringing until it eventually slows to a stop. If one were to grab the bell while it was ringing, or wrap it in a heavy blanket, it would markedly decrease the length of the ringing of the bell. In pulsed-wave ultrasound, short pulses are very desirable; anything that will decrease the length of the pulse improves the axial resolution of the image (Figure 2-9). Damping decreases the number of cycles in a pulse, effectively decreasing the **spatial pulse length** (SPL). Damping shortens the pulse to 2 or 3 cycles per pulse.

Other Effects of Damping

Although damping in general has its advantages, there are also some side effects of damping (Table 2-4). One of these side effects is decreased **sensitivity**

FIGURE 2-9 Damping. Ultrasound pulse with light damping produces many cycles in a pulse **(A)**. With heavy damping, the number of cycles in the pulse is reduced, shortening the pulse **(B)**. (Image reprinted with permission from Bushberg J. The Essential Physics of Medical Imaging. 2nd Ed. Philadelphia, PA: Lippincott Williams & Wilkins, 2002:487.)

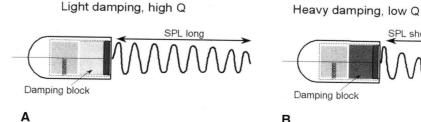

Light damping, high Q

SPL long

Damping block

Heavy damping, low Q

SPL short

Damping block

A   **B**

TABLE 2-4 Side effects of damping. *Note:* these are not necessarily all bad side effects. For example, increased bandwidth and a low quality factor are good side effects.
Side Effects of Damping
Decreases sensitivity of the transducer Increases the bandwidth Reduces the quality factor

of the transducer. Sensitivity is the ability of a system to display low-level or weak echoes. Another side effect of damping is the production of other frequencies in the beam in addition to the operating frequency. **Bandwidth** is the range of frequencies present within the beam. Essentially, damping produces a "less pure" operating frequency. Continuous-wave (CW) transducers do not have any damping. Therefore, if a sample of the beam of a 4.0-MHz CW transducer is taken, a 4.0-MHz beam will be discovered. However, once damping is applied, as with pulsed-wave transducers, the beam loses its purity. That is, if a sample of the beam of a 4.0-MHz pulsed-wave transducer were obtained, many frequencies would be present in addition to the 4.0-MHz center frequency. This wide range of frequencies is the bandwidth of the transducer.

The more damping there is, the shorter the pulse and the wider the bandwidth (Figure 2-10). The **quality factor** (Q-factor) is a term used to quantitate the purity of the beam. The Q-factor is the operating frequency of the transducer divided by the bandwidth (Table 2-5). Pulsed-wave transducers have typically low Q-factors because they need damping to make the pulse

FIGURE 2-10 Bandwidth. This diagram demonstrates the relationship between pulse duration, or length, and bandwidth. With increasing pulse length, the bandwidth becomes narrower, thereby reducing resolution. Therefore, to improve resolution, a short pulse length should be employed. (Image reprinted with permission from Feigenbaum H. Feigenbaum's Echocardiography. 6th Ed. Philadelphia, PA: Lippincott Williams & Wilkins, 2004.)

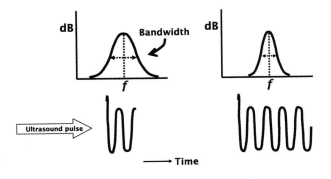

As pulse length increases, the frequency spectrum narrows
∴ Longer pulse length ⇒ narrower bandwidth ⇒ lower resolution

TABLE 2-5 Formula for the quality factor. Quality factor is determined by dividing the operating frequency (F_o) by the bandwidth. *Note:* "Q" stands for "quality." However, it is not the resolution of the image that is being referred to when the word "quality factor" is used, but the purity of the beam. The question should be asked "How near to the actual operating frequency is the bandwidth?"
Formula
$$\text{Q-factor} = \frac{F_o}{\text{Bandwidth}}$$

FIGURE 2-11 Quality factor (Q-factor). Continuous-wave probes are not damped, so they have a high Q-factor **(A)**. With pulse-wave probes **(B,C)**, the more damping there is (signified by the gray boxes within the transducers shown in B & C), the shorter the pulse, and therefore, the wider the bandwidth and lower the Q-factor.

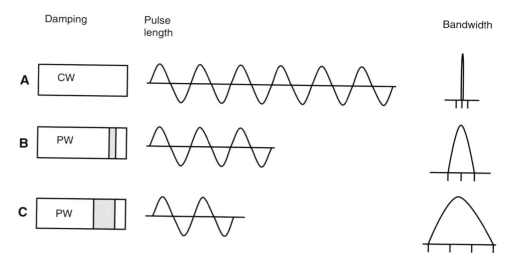

TABLE 2 - 6 Summary of the effects of damping on the pulse. *Note:* The aim of damping is to obtain the finest diagnostic image with the best axial resolution.
↑ Damping = ↓ Spatial pulse length = ↑ Bandwidth = ↓ Q-factor = Better axial resolution

short. CW transducers have a narrow bandwidth as a result of the absence of a backing material, with subsequent high Q-factors (Figure 2-11 and Table 2-6).

REAL-TIME SCANNING

Modern ultrasound equipment utilizes **real-time**, or **automatic scanning**, to obtain diagnostic images of the body. With real-time scanning, the transducer is responsible for sending out **scan lines** across a defined plane. Images are produced when an ultrasound beam is swept across that plane. Pulses of ultrasound are sent out and produce scan lines. All of the scan lines, when placed next to each other, form an image that is called a **frame**.

TYPES OF TRANSDUCERS

There are two methods of sending out scan lines to form an image using real-time: mechanical scanning (via mechanical transducers) and electronic scanning (via electronic transducers). Both of these methods provide a means for sweeping the ultrasound beam through the tissue repeatedly and rapidly. While electronic scanning is most often the method employed today, a brief review of mechanical transducers will be provided in the next section.

Mechanical Transducers

Mechanical scanheads are not commonly utilized in today's busy sonography departments. These transducers typically had one or more piezoelectric elements connected to a motor, or a fixed element with a mirror connected to

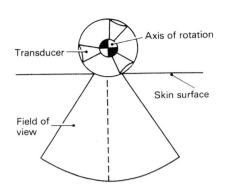

FIGURE 2-12 Mechanical sector scanner. (Image reprinted with permission from Sanders R. Clinical Sonography: A Practical Guide. 4th Ed. Philadelphia, PA: Lippincott Williams & Wilkins, 2007:10.)

a motor (Figure 2-12). The motor steered the element, or a mirror, to produce the scan lines that made up the image. This produced a sector image pattern. The piezoelectric element and motor were inside of a protective housing. Oil was used as a coupling medium to prevent air from forming within the housing. Air within the housing would hamper the transmission of the sound. These transducers were fixed frequency and fixed focus. That is, in order to change the frequency or the location of the focal zone, one had to change the entire scanhead. Focusing of the beam was achieved by either the shape of the element or the use of a lens. The major advantages of the mechanical transducer were that they were inexpensive and typically had a small **footprint**. Unfortunately, they were fragile and their mechanical elements were easily broken.

Electronic Transducers

Electronic scanning is performed with transducers that have multiple active elements. This is referred to as an **array**. An array is formed by taking a single slab of PZT and slicing it down into multiple subelements. Each subelement is connected to a wire, so it may fire independently (Figure 2-7). The system can selectively excite the elements as needed to shape and steer the beam. With most array transducers, no motors are needed for beam steering. Arrays may be either sequenced or phased and can produce various image shapes.

Linear Sequenced Array
The **linear sequenced array**, also referred to as the linear sequential array or linear array, is a transducer that is often used in vascular or small parts imaging (Figure 2-13). This transducer produces a rectangular shaped image

FIGURE 2-13 Linear sequenced array transducer. **A.** The image footprint of the linear sequenced array transducer. **B.** Image of a linear sequenced array transducer. (Image reprinted with permission from Cosby KS. Practical Guide to Emergency Ultrasound. Philadelphia, PA: Lippincott Williams & Wilkins, 2005.)

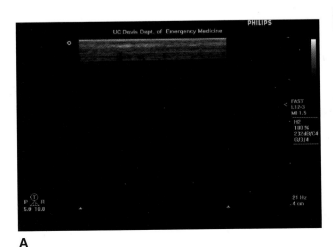

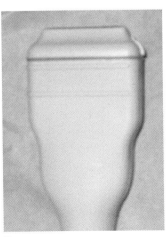

A

B

FIGURE 2-14 Linear sequenced array transducer format **(left)** and image **(right)**. (Image reprinted with permission from Brant W. Ultrasound. Philadelphia, PA: Lippincott Williams & Wilkins, 2001:2.)

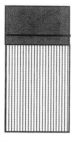

Linear array

A

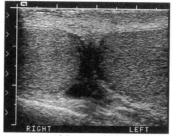

Linear array

B

T A B L E   2 - 7   Linear sequenced array.
Linear Sequenced Array
• Also referred to as linear sequential array or linear array
• Rectangular shaped image
• Firing is sequenced
• Electronic steering available
• Electronically focused
• Used for vascular and small parts imaging

(Figure 2-14). With the linear sequenced array, the elements are arranged in a line, next to each other, but are fired in small groups in sequence. For example, the elements are not fired 1–2–3–4–5 but are fired (1–2–3) . . . (4–5–6) . . . (7–8–9). Linear sequenced arrays do not need any beam steering to produce a rectangular image. However, should beam steering be needed, whether for Doppler or to create a vector image, the beam can be electronically steered (Table 2-7).

Curved Sequenced Array

The **curved sequenced array** transducer, also referred to as a convex, curvilinear, or curved sequential array, is based on the same technology as that of the linear sequenced array but with a curved face (Figures 2-15 and 2-16). As with the linear sequenced array, the elements are fired in groups (Table 2-8).

FIGURE 2-15 Curvilinear array transducer. **A.** The image footprint of the curvilinear array transducer. **B.** Image of a curvilinear array transducer. (Image reprinted with permission from Cosby KS. Practical Guide to Emergency Ultrasound. Philadelphia, PA: Lippincott Williams & Wilkins, 2005.)

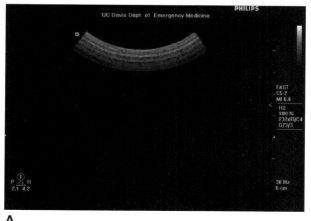

A

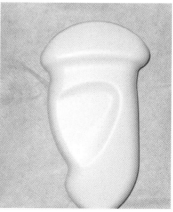

B

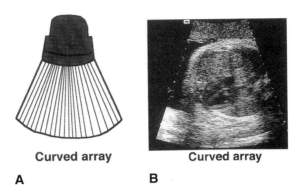

FIGURE 2-16 Curved sequenced array transducer format **(A)** and image **(B)**. (Image reprinted with permission from Brant W. Ultrasound. Philadelphia, PA: Lippincott Williams & Wilkins, 2001:2.)

T A B L E **2 - 8** Curved sequenced array.
Curved Sequenced Array
• Also referred to as a convex, curvilinear, or curved sequential array
• Curved shape image
• Firing is sequenced
• Electronically focused
• Used for abdominal, gynecology, and obstetrics imaging

Linear Phased Arrays

The **linear phased array**, also referred to as simply a phased array, is more commonly known as a sector or vector transducer (Figure 2-17). This probe typically has a small footprint and is used for cardiac imaging, neonatal brain imaging, with some endocavitary transducers, and any other application where a sector image shape is desired (Figure 2-18).

The phased array transducer has a small footprint. In order to create a sector image, electronic steering is needed for every scan line. Unlike the curved and linear sequenced arrays, where the shape of the transducer dictates the shape of the image, in the phased array the shape of the face of the

FIGURE 2-17 Linear phased array transducer. This phased array transducer **(A)** will yield a sector shaped image **(B)**. (Image reprinted with permission from Cosby KS. Practical Guide to Emergency Ultrasound. Philadelphia, PA: Lippincott Williams & Wilkins, 2005.)

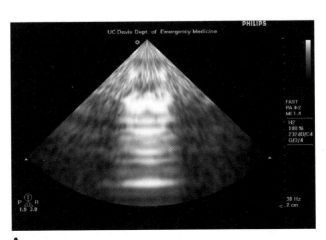

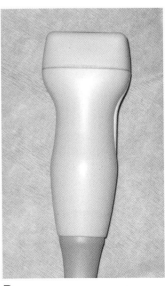

FIGURE 2-18 Endovaginal transducer. This is a type of a phased array transducer. (Image reprinted with permission from Sanders R. Clinical Sonography: A Practical Guide. 4th Ed. Philadelphia, PA: Lippincott Williams & Wilkins, 2007:13.)

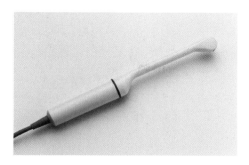

FIGURE 2-19 Phased array transducer and sector versus vector image shapes. **A.** A sector transducer produces a "piece of pie"-shaped image with a common point of origin on the transducer face. **B.** Vector transducers are sector transducers in which the scan lines do not have a common point of origin. (Image reprinted with permission from Brant W. Ultrasound. Philadelphia, PA: Lippincott Williams & Wilkins, 2001:2.)

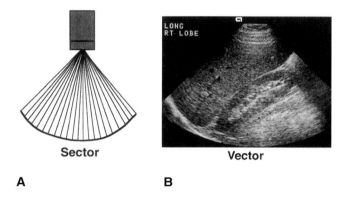

transducer does not resemble the shape of the image. This transducer can take either the sector, or true "pie-shaped" image, or the vector image shape, which is the flat-topped, trapezoidal image shape (Figure 2-19).

Naturally, the phased array uses **phasing** to steer and focus the beam (Table 2-9). Phasing is changing the timing of the shocking of the elements in order to shape and steer the beam. All arrays are phased focused. That is, all of the array transducers mentioned in this section use phasing to control the focusing in the scan plane. Phasing provides the sonographer the ability to control the depth of the focal zone in the scan plane. The order in which the elements are shocked determines beam steering and focusing (Figures 2-20 to 2-22).

Annular Array

The annular array, which is not currently being produced, is the only array that is mechanically steered (Figure 2-23). It is phased focused, but the steering is performed with a motor. The transducer is made up of one disc-shaped

TABLE 2-9 Linear phased array.
Linear Phased Array
• Also referred to as phased arrays, sector, or vector transducer
• Vector or sector shaped image
• Electronic steering and focusing by phasing
• Used for cardiac, abdominal, neonatal imaging, and endocavity transducers

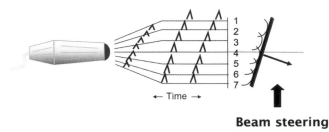

Beam steering

FIGURE 2-20 Phasing and beam steering. Phased array technology permits steering of the ultrasound beam. By adjusting the timing of excitation of the individual piezoelectric crystals, the wavefront of ultrasound energy can be directed, as shown. Beam steering is a fundamental feature of how two-dimensional images are created. (Image reprinted with permission from Feigenbaum H. Feigenbaum's Echocardiography. 6th Ed. Philadelphia, PA: Lippincott Williams & Wilkins, 2004.)

FIGURE 2-21 Beam steering. The beam former electronically steers the beam by introducing phase delays during the transmit and receive timing of the phased array transducer. (Image reprinted with permission from Bushberg J. The Essential Physics of Medical Imaging. 2nd Ed. Philadelphia, PA: Lippincott Williams & Wilkins, 2002:513.)

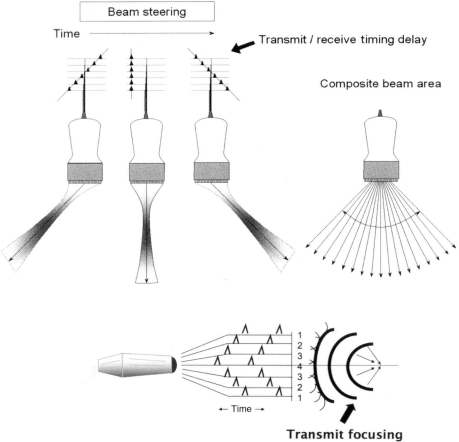

FIGURE 2-22 Phasing and focusing. By adjusting the timing of excitation of the individual crystals within a phased array transducer, the beam can be focused. In this example, the outer elements are fired first, followed sequentially by the more central elements. Because the speed of sound is fixed, this manipulation in the timing of excitation results in a wavefront that is curved and focused. This is called "transmit focusing." Changing the timing of when the elements are shocked focuses the beam. (Image reprinted with permission from Feigenbaum H. Feigenbaum's Echocardiography. 6th Ed. Philadelphia, PA: Lippincott Williams & Wilkins, 2004.)

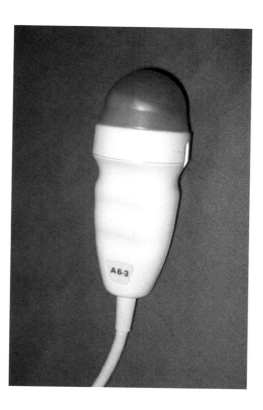

FIGURE 2-23   Annular array. The annular array is mechanically steered (with a motor) and electronically focused.

element cut into concentric circles. Each circle of the "bulls-eye" is wired to act independently. The advantage to this transducer is that it has excellent lateral resolution. The annular array produces a sector image (Table 2-10).

Three-Dimensional Transducers

Three-dimensional (3D) ultrasound images are traditionally made up of two-dimensional (2D) acquisitions placed next to each other. There are three different ways to create the 3D image: freehand, with a mechanical transducer, or the newest method, electronically, with the latest 2D array technology.

In the freehand method, also referred to as manual, the sonographer is responsible for moving the transducer through a path to gather the 2D slices. This method is the most operator dependent, as it relies upon the steady hand of the sonographer to move the transducer at the same speed over the tissue. Because of the potential variability in movement across the plane, measurements of the 3D image are not possible with freehand 3D technique. The 2D slices, once converted to 3D format, may then be sliced to view coronal, sagittal, and axial planes. With the mechanical technique, also referred to as automated or mechanical 3D method, specialized transducers have been developed that are essentially curved sequenced array

T A B L E 2 - 1 0   Annular array.
Annular Array
• Mechanically steered
• Electronically focused by phasing
• Sector shaped image

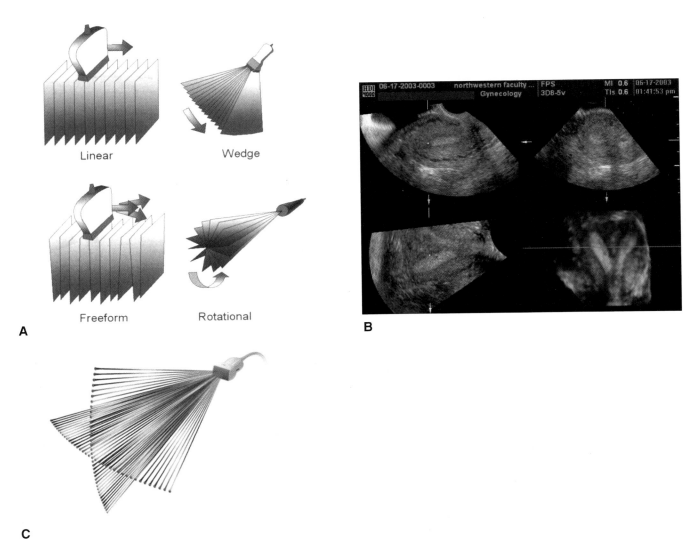

FIGURE 2-24 Three-dimensional imaging. **A.** Different ways of obtaining 3D image. **B.** 3D multiplanar image. (Image reprinted with permission from Baggish M. The Essential Physics of Medical Imaging. 2nd Ed. Philadelphia, PA: Lippincott Williams & Wilkins, 2002:524.) **C.** 2D transducer capable of capturing real-time volumes with no motor needed for steering the beam (courtesy Philips Healthcare).

transducers mounted onto a motor. These transducers permit measurement on the screen of the 3D image as well as the use of real-time 3D, also known as four-dimensional (4D) ultrasound. The **frame rate** of the 4D image is limited by the speed of the motor to which the transducer is attached. The latest technology for acquiring a 3D image is the new electronic array, called a 2D transducer. These transducers acquire real-time volumes using transducers with greater than 2500 elements (Figure 2-24).

Continuous-Wave Transducers

CW transducers are most often utilized in Doppler studies. A dedicated CW transducer will contain two piezoelectric elements: one to continuously transmit sound and one to continuously receive sound. No image is generated with these transducers, because it is not possible to time how long it takes the echoes to return (Figure 2-25).

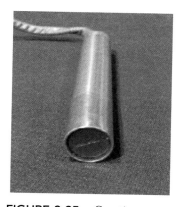

FIGURE 2-25 Continuous-wave transducer. A continuous-wave transducer uses two elements: one for producing sound and one for receiving sound.

RESOLUTION

Spatial Resolution

Spatial resolution can be defined as the ability of the system to distinguish between closely spaced objects. Spatial (meaning space) resolution relates to the quality of the detail of the image. It can be divided into four components: **axial resolution**, **lateral resolution**, **elevational resolution**, and **contrast resolution** (Table 2-11 and Figure 2-26).

Axial Resolution

Axial resolution is the minimum distance two reflectors can be, parallel to the beam, and still appear on the screen as two dots. That is, if the transducer is aiming at two reflectors on the screen (parallel to the beam), then two dots should appear on the display (Figure 2-27). Axial resolution may also be referred to as longitudinal, axial, radial, range, and depth. Remembering the word "LARRD" can help one recall the different names for axial resolution (Table 2-11).

TABLE 2-11 Spatial resolution.		
Components of Spatial Resolution	**Definition**	**Synonyms**
Axial resolution	The minimum distance two reflectors can be, parallel to the beam, and still appear on the screen as two dots	Longitudinal Axial Radial Range Depth
Lateral resolution	The ability to accurately identify reflectors that are arranged perpendicular to the ultrasound beam	Lateral Angular Transverse Azimuthal
Elevational resolution	The resolution in the third dimension of the beam: the slice-thickness plane	Slice- or section-thickness plane resolution
Contrast resolution	The ability to differentiate one shade of gray from another	None

FIGURE 2-26 Primary determinants of axial, lateral, contrast, and temporal resolution. (Image reprinted with permission from Feigenbaum H. Feigenbaum's Echocardiography. 6th Ed. Philadelphia, PA: Lippincott Williams & Wilkins, 2004.)

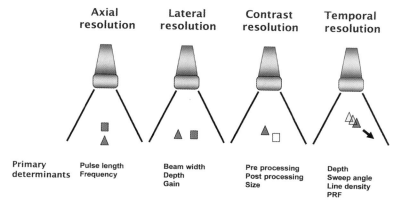

FIGURE 2-27 Axial resolution. Axial resolution is the minimum distance two reflectors can be, parallel to the beam, and still appear on the screen as two dots. In **(A)**, a transducer (TD) with a low-frequency beam is aiming at two reflectors in soft tissue. This beam has a relatively long spatial pulse length (SPL), so only one return echo is generated as a result of encountering the two reflectors. In **(B)**, a TD with a higher-frequency beam is aiming at the same two reflectors in soft tissue. This beam has relatively short SPL; therefore, it generates return echoes from both reflectors independently.

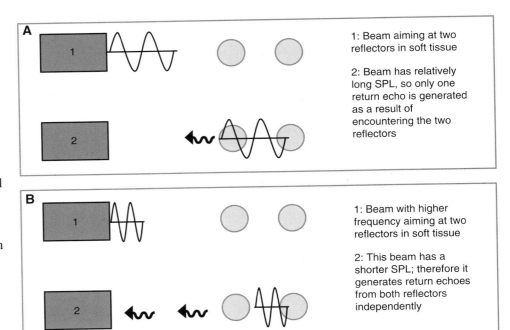

A
1: Beam aiming at two reflectors in soft tissue

2: Beam has relatively long SPL, so only one return echo is generated as a result of encountering the two reflectors

B
1: Beam with higher frequency aiming at two reflectors in soft tissue

2: This beam has a shorter SPL; therefore it generates return echoes from both reflectors independently

The spatial pulse length determines the system's axial resolution. Specifically, the shorter the pulse used, the better the axial resolution of the system. The system decreases the length of the pulse by either decreasing the wavelength or decreasing the number of cycles per pulse (Table 2-12). The number of cycles can be decreased by adding more damping material. The wavelength can be decreased by increasing the frequency (Table 2-13). Therefore, increasing the frequency shortens the pulse, which is why higher-frequency transducers offer better axial resolution than lower-frequency transducers (Figure 2-28). Axial resolution is equal to one half the SPL (Table 2-14). It is important to note that if the SPL decreases, the numerical value for axial resolution decreases. Therefore, the lower the numerical value for axial resolution, the better the axial resolution of the transducer. That is to say, that an axial resolution of 0.2 mm is better than an axial resolution of 0.4 mm because two reflectors could be as close as 0.2 mm apart

TABLE 2-12 Spatial pulse length. Spatial pulse length (SPL) is equal to the wavelength (λ) multiplied by the number of cycles (n) in the pulse.
Formula
$SPL = \lambda n$

TABLE 2-13 Wavelength. Wavelength (λ) is equal to the propagation speed (c) divided by the frequency (f).
Formula
$\lambda = \dfrac{c}{f}$

FIGURE 2-28 Frequency and axial resolution. The axial resolution of a high-frequency transducer **(A)** is much better at identifying separate pins *(arrow)* compared with the axial resolution of a lower-frequency transducer **(B)**, in which the pins merge and appear less distinct.

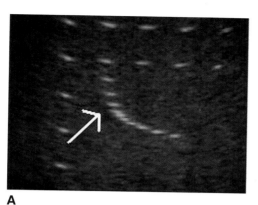

A

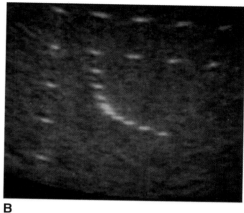

B

and still be resolved as two distinct echoes. Some examples of questions that may be asked about axial resolution are provided in Table 2-15.

Lateral Resolution

While axial resolution is the minimum distance two reflectors can be, parallel to the beam, and still appear on the screen as two dots, lateral resolution relates to the width of the beam and the reflectors that lie perpendicular to it (Figure 2-29). Lateral resolution may also be referred to as lateral, angular, transverse, and azimuthal. Remembering the word "LATA" can help one recall the different names for axial resolution (Table 2-11). Poor lateral resolution occurs when reflectors appear to be wider than they are supposed to be (Figure 2-30).

TABLE 2-14 Axial resolution. The axial resolution is equal to one half the spatial pulse length (SPL).

Formula
Axial resolution = ½ SPL

TABLE 2-15 Examples of questions relating to axial resolution.

Question	Explanation
The axial resolution of the transducer distance is 0.2 mm. What is the smallest two reflectors can be in order to appear as two echoes on the screen?	The answer is 0.2 mm. The two reflectors have to be the same as the axial resolution of the transducer or greater in order to be displayed as two distinct echoes.
The spatial pulse length of the transducer is 0.2 mm. What is the smallest distance two reflectors can be in order to appear as two echoes on the screen?	The answer is 0.1 mm. This time the SPL is given, not the axial resolution. The axial resolution of a transducer equals ½ SPL, so the SPL has to be halved in order to determine the axial resolution. In this case, ½ SPL = 0.1 mm.

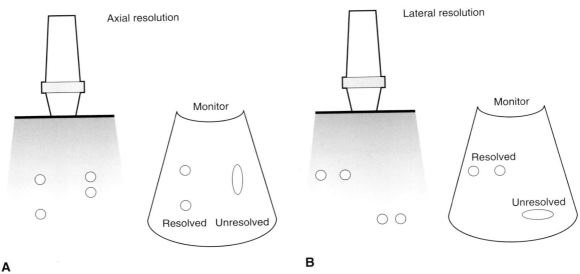

FIGURE 2-29 Difference between axial and lateral resolution. Axial resolution is in line with the scanning plane **(A)**. Lateral resolution is perpendicular to the scanning plane **(B)**. (Image reprinted with permission from Cosby KS. Practical Guide to Emergency Ultrasound. Philadelphia, PA: Lippincott Williams & Wilkins, 2005.)

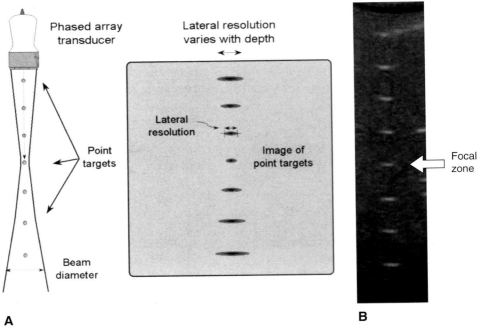

FIGURE 2-30 Lateral resolution. The beam changes shape as it travels deeper **(A)**. Depending on where the reflectors are located in the beam determines the lateral resolution. **(B)** Notice how the reflectors appear to be wider where the beam diverges in this sonographic image of a tissue equivalent phantom showing lateral resolution. (Image reprinted with permission from Bushberg J. The Essential Physics of Medical Imaging. 2nd Ed. Philadelphia, PA: Lippincott Williams & Wilkins, 2002:499.)

FIGURE 2-31 Hourglass-shaped ultrasound beam. Near field (zone) and far field (zone) (Image reprinted with permission from Bushberg J. The Essential Physics of Medical Imaging. 2nd Ed. Philadelphia, PA: Lippincott Williams & Wilkins, 2002:231.)

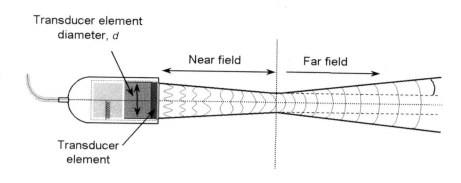

The diameter of the beam is determined by both the frequency and the diameter of the element itself, also referred to as the **aperture**. The beam takes on a shape in the appearance of an hourglass (Figure 2-31). As the beam leaves the transducer and travels into the patient, the diameter of the beam varies with distance. The beam begins to narrow immediately upon leaving the transducer. At its narrowest point, it is called the **focal point**. The region from the transducer face to the focal point is called the **near zone** or **Fresnel zone**. Subsequently, the length of the near zone is referred to as the **near zone length** (NZL). After the focal point is reached, the beam starts to diverge, or spread. The region distal to the focal point is called the **far zone** or **Fraunhofer zone**. **Divergence**, or the spreading out of the beam, which is the result of diffraction, is detrimental to lateral resolution. Recall that a narrow beam width is desired in order to have good lateral resolution. Subsequently, the focal zone should be placed at or below the area of interest to obtain the best lateral resolution in that area.

Unfocused transducers have a natural focal zone. Assuming an unfocused beam from a single-element transducer, the beam diameter has several specific characteristics (Table 2-16 and Figure 2-32). As the beam propagates, its diameter changes. Therefore, lateral resolution does vary with depth. Both the actual diameter of the element and the frequency of the transducer have an effect on the NZL and the amount of divergence in the far field. A smaller aperture results in a shorter NZL and more divergence in the far field. If the transducer and the frequency do not change, but a larger aperture is utilized, a longer NZL will result, with less divergence in the far field. The same theory is true for identical aperture size, but different frequencies. That is, for a given aperture, the lower the frequency, the shorter the NZL, with an increase of divergence in the far field. Conversely, the

TABLE 2-16 Characteristics of an unfocused single-element transducer.
Characteristics of an Unfocused Single-Element Transducer
• At the face of the transducer, the beam diameter is equal to the element diameter.
• At a distance of one near zone length, the beam diameter is equal to one half of the diameter of the element.
• At a distance of two near zone lengths, the beam diameter again equals the element diameter.

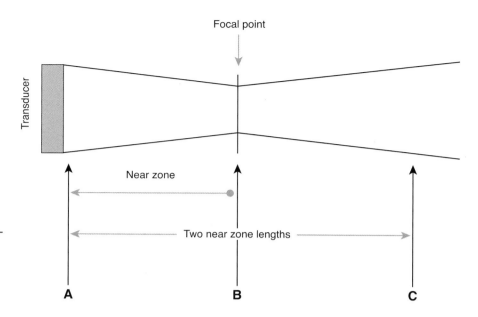

FIGURE 2-32 Single-element unfocused transducer. At the face of the transducer **(A)**, the beam width equals the element diameter. At a distance of one near-zone length **(B)**, the beam diameter is half the element diameter. At a distance of two near-zone lengths **(C)**, the beam diameter again equals the element diameter. Deep to this point, the beam continues to diverge.

higher the frequency, the longer the NZL, with less divergence in the far field (Table 2-17). As with axial resolution, the smaller the numerical value for lateral resolution, the better. Therefore, a lateral resolution of 0.2 mm is better than a lateral resolution of 0.4 mm. It is important to note that most transducers have better axial resolution than lateral resolution.

Elevational Resolution and Contrast Resolution

An ultrasound image is a 2D representation of 3D objects. The image seen on the ultrasound monitor is flat. However, the ultrasound beam is not razor thin. The beam has a definite thickness. The image on the ultrasound monitor is a compressed version of any object located within the ultrasound beam. Therefore, bogus echoes may be seen within a simple cyst because the beam is also slicing through the tissue next to the cyst. This third dimension of the beam is called the **slice-thickness plane**. The slice-thickness plane may also be referred to as the **section-thickness plane** or the **elevational plane**. Elevational resolution is the resolution in the third dimension of the beam.

In order to obtain the most diagnostic representation of the body, the thinnest plane possible must be utilized. As with lateral resolution, the thinnest elevational plane is optimal. This is achieved by focusing. However, unlike electronic transducers with phased focusing, most transducers are still focused mechanically, with a lens, in the slice-thickness plane. Because the slice-thickness plane is focused with a lens, the focus is fixed and does not change regardless of the depth (Figure 2-33).

T A B L E 2 - 17 The relationship between frequency, aperture size, near zone length (NZL), and divergence in the far field.

Adjustment	Result
↑ Frequency	↑ NZL and ↓ divergence in far field
↑ Aperture	↑ NZL and ↓ divergence in far field

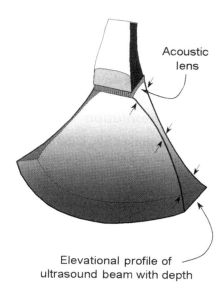

FIGURE 2-33 Elevational resolution. Elevational resolution is most commonly focused with a lens. (Image reprinted with permission from Bushberg J. The Essential Physics of Medical Imaging. 2nd Ed. Philadelphia, PA: Lippincott Williams & Wilkins, 2002:497.)

Transducers with the latest technology have the ability to focus electronically in the elevational plane (Figure 2-34). These transducers are often referred to as 1.5D transducers. These transducers automatically change the slice-thickness focal zone when the focal zone is changed by the operator. **Contrast resolution** the ability to differentiate one shade of gray from another. It is related to dynamic range, which is discussed further in Chapter 3 of this book.

Temporal Resolution

Temporal resolution represents time, or the ability to display structures in real time. Temporal resolution, or time resolution, relates to how quickly frames are generated. Another, more commonly used term for temporal resolution is frame rate. A complete ultrasound image, or frame, needs to be placed on the screen, scan line by scan line, before the next frame can

FIGURE 2-34 A 1.5D transducer. The 1.5D transducer is capable of electronically focusing the beam in the elevational plane. (Image reprinted with permission from Bushberg J. The Essential Physics of Medical Imaging. 2nd Ed. Philadelphia, PA: Lippincott Williams & Wilkins, 2002:500.)

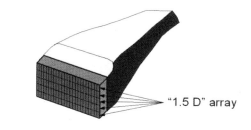

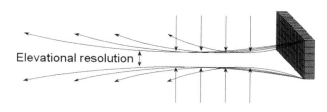

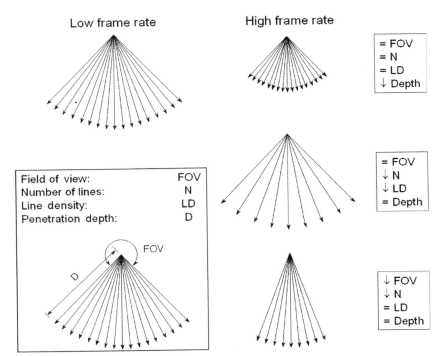

Low frame rate   High frame rate

- = FOV
- = N
- = LD
- ↓ Depth

Field of view: FOV
Number of lines: N
Line density: LD
Penetration depth: D

FOV

D

- = FOV
- ↓ N
- ↓ LD
- = Depth

- ↓ FOV
- ↓ N
- = LD
- = Depth

FIGURE 2-35   Temporal resolution and frame rate. Temporal resolution represents time, or the ability to display structures in real time. Ultrasound image quality depends on several factors, including the field of view (FOV), the number of scan lines per image (N), the line density (LD), and penetration depth (D) **(inset)**, in addition to the image frame rate. Preserving the frame rate involves trade-offs. Changing anyone of the aforementioned parameters will affect the frame rate unless something else is changed to counter the effect. For example, if the depth is decreased, the frame rate will increase **(top right)**. If the depth is then increased, however, in order to preserve the frame rate either the line density or field of view must decrease **(middle and lower right)**. (Image reprinted with permission from Bushberg J. The Essential Physics of Medical Imaging. 2nd Ed. Philadelphia, PA: Lippincott Williams & Wilkins, 2002:514.)

begin to be placed. The longer it takes a frame to be displayed on the screen, the lower the frame rate, and the worse the temporal resolution. The unit in which frame rate can be expressed is either hertz, or frames per second. A minimum frame rate of 15 Hz needs to be maintained or the image will flicker.

There are three adjustments that can be made to alter the frame rate in grayscale imaging: image depth (PRF), the number of focal zones, and the number of scan lines per frame or line density (Figure 2-35). As the depth is increased, the pulse has to travel farther or deeper into the body. A new pulse cannot be sent out until the previous pulse is received. Therefore, the machine has to wait before sending out the next pulse. The longer it takes to create one scan line, the longer it takes to display one frame. Therefore, PRF is directly related to frame rate. That is, the higher the PRF, and therefore, the more shallow the image, the higher the frame rate. Recall that focal zones are created by phasing. However, there can only be one focal zone per scan line. If more than one focal zone is desired, it will take an extra pulse per scan line for each focal zone desired.

TABLE 2-18 Formula for frame rate. The frame rate (FR) is equal to the pulse repetition frequency (PRF) divided by the lines per frame (LPF).
Formula
$$FR = \dfrac{PRF}{LPF}$$

The latest ultrasound technology allows the width of the image to be increased or decreased. The more scan lines that need to be displayed, the longer it takes to create one frame, and therefore, the worse the temporal resolution. A wider image will usually require more scan lines than a narrower image. In the instance where the temporal resolution is inadequate, such as imaging a deep structure while using multiple focal zones, the frame rate can be improved by using a narrower image width, thereby decreasing the number of lines per frame. The frame rate is equal to the PRF divided by the lines per frame (Table 2-18).

TRANSDUCER CARE AND MAINTENANCE

Proper handling of the transducer is essential in order to prevent damage to the cord, connector, and piezoelectric elements. Transducers should be hung in the proper transducer holder on the equipment and never dangled over the handle of the machine. Hanging the transducer improperly places undue stress on the cord and may damage the wires inside. Likewise, dangling the transducer over the machine handle increases the risk of the transducer falling to the ground and potentially causing permanent and irreparable damage. Both the transducer and the power cords should be carefully draped so as to avoid rolling the machine over the cord as well. When the cord or probe is damaged, it may appear on the screen as an area of dropout (Figure 2-36).

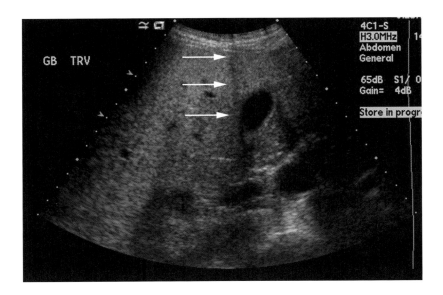

FIGURE 2-36 Tranducer damage. An area of dropout *(arrows)* can be noted within this image.

REVIEW QUESTIONS

1. Which of the following would be considered the narrowest part of a sound beam?
   a. Far zone
   b. Near zone
   c. Near zone length
   d. Focus

2. Which of the following is the part of the transducer that stops the ringing of the element?
   a. Matching layer
   b. Housing
   c. Damping material
   d. Insulator

3. Along with image depth, which of the following also determines the frame rate?
   a. Axial resolution
   b. Frequency
   c. Number of lines per frame
   d. Lateral resolution

4. Which type of resolution is an accurate representation of moving structures?
   a. Lateral resolution
   b. Azimuthal resolution
   c. Spatial resolution
   d. Temporal resolution

5. Which of the following is the type of transducer that utilizes elements arranged in a concentric pattern?
   a. Phased array
   b. Annular array
   c. Mechanical
   d. Linear

6. Which of the following would be considered an advantage of a curved linear array over a phased array transducer?
   a. Wider near field
   b. Linear scan lines
   c. Narrower near field
   d. Narrower far field

7. Which of the following is not a true statement about a mechanical transducer?
   a. It uses a motor to steer the beam
   b. Most transducers are no longer mechanical
   c. May be focused with a lens or phased focused
   d. There are no moving parts

8. Along with crystal diameter, the divergence in the far field is also determined by which of the following?
   a. Spatial Pulse Length
   b. Frequency
   c. Propagation speed
   d. Line density

9. Which of the following would cause a decrease in temporal resolution?
   a. Increased line density
   b. Decreased sector size
   c. Single transmit zone
   d. Decreased line density

10. Which of the following would cause an increase in frame rate?
    a. Multifocusing
    b. Increased line density
    c. Increased imaging depth
    d. Decreased imaging depth

11. Which of the following is true of the diameter of the sound beam in the Fresnel zone?
    a. It increases
    b. It decreases
    c. It does not change
    d. It is unpredictable

12. Which resolution is best in clinical imaging?
    a. Axial
    b. Lateral
    c. Temporal
    d. Slice thickness

13. Which of the following will increase the near zone length?
    a. Large crystal diameter, low frequency
    b. Small crystal diameter, low frequency
    c. Large crystal diameter, high frequency
    d. Small crystal diameter, high frequency

14. Which of the following will decrease beam divergence in the far field?
    a. Large crystal diameter, low frequency
    b. Small crystal diameter, low frequency
    c. Large crystal diameter, high frequency
    d. Small crystal diameter, high frequency

15. Imaging transducers have:
    a. Low quality factors, wide bandwidths
    b. High quality factors, narrow bandwidths
    c. Low quality factors, narrow bandwidths
    d. High quality factors, wide bandwidths

16. Damping material produces all of the following except:
    a. Decreased sensitivity
    b. Increased SPL
    c. Wide bandwidths
    d. Low quality factors

17. Which of the following electrical patterns produces electronic focusing of the ultrasound beam?
    a. Curve
    b. Slope
    c. Width
    d. Length

18. In an unfocused, single-element transducer, the focal point of the sound beam measures how much of the total beam width?
    a. One fourth
    b. One third
    c. One half
    d. Equal

19. Which of the following facilitates the transmission of sound from the element into the patient's skin?
    a. Damping material
    b. Matching layer
    c. Tungsten covering
    d. Focusing material

20. Which of the following is the range of frequencies present within the beam?
    a. Quality factor
    b. Bandwidth
    c. Array
    d. Wavefront

21. Which type of interference results in a larger sound wave?
    a. Constructive interference
    b. Destructive interference
    c. True interference
    d. False interference

22. Which of the following transducers uses a motor for steering the beam?
    a. Linear phased array
    b. Sequential linear array
    c. Mechanical transducer
    d. Curvilinear sequenced array

23. Which of the following best describes the components of the damping material?
    a. Epoxy resin loaded with tungsten
    b. Tungsten resin loaded with lead zirconate titanate
    c. Lead zirconate titanate impregnated with tungsten
    d. Tungsten impregnated with lead

24. Which of the following is not true of the linear sequenced array transducer?
    a. Rectangular shape image
    b. Firing is sequenced
    c. Electronically focused
    d. The elements are arranged in a ring

25. Which of the following is not a true statement?
    a. Lateral resolution varies with depth
    b. A larger aperture results in a shorter near zone length
    c. A larger aperture produces less divergence in the far field
    d. Lateral resolution may also be referred to as azimuthal resolution

26. Which of the following is not true of damping?
    a. Damping decreases the number of cycles in a pulse
    b. Damping decreases spatial pulse length
    c. Damping worsens axial resolution
    d. Damping decreases the sensitivity of the transducer

27. Which of the following is not a synonym for axial resolution?
    a. Angular
    b. Range
    c. Depth
    d. Radial

28. Temporal resolution relates to which of the following?
    a. Lateral resolution
    b. Frame rate
    c. Range ambiguity
    d. Element diameter

29. Which of the following may also be referred to as the far zone?
    a. Frame zone
    b. Fresnel zone
    c. Fraunhofer zone
    d. Frankincense zone

30. What states that waves are the result of the interference of many wavelets produced at the face of the transducer?
    a. Curie's principle
    b. Snell's law
    c. Bernoulli's law
    d. Huygen's principle

31. Which of the following is the resolution in the third dimension of the beam?
    a. Lateral resolution
    b. Elevational resolution
    c. Contrast resolution
    d. Longitudinal resolution

32. Which of the following is true concerning the frequency and the near zone length?
    a. The higher the frequency, the longer the near zone length
    b. The lower the frequency, the longer the near zone length
    c. Frequency and near zone length are not related
    d. Frequency and near zone length cannot be adjusted

33. Which of the following is defined as changing the timing of the shocking of the elements in order to shape and steer the beam?
    a. Angulation
    b. Focusing
    c. Phasing
    d. Bundling

34. Which of the following is not a component of spatial resolution?
    a. Frame resolution
    b. Contrast resolution
    c. Axial resolution
    d. Elevational resolution

35. Which types of transducers are no longer used?
    a. Continuous-wave transducers
    b. Curved sequenced array transducers
    c. Linear sequenced array transducers
    d. Annular array transducers

36. Which of the following transducers is not used for imaging?
    a. Continuous-wave transducers
    b. Curved sequenced array transducers
    c. Linear sequenced array transducers
    d. Annular array transducers

37. Which of the following transducers is also referred to as a sector or vector transducer?
    a. Linear sequential array
    b. Linear phased array
    c. Continuous-wave transducer
    d. Curved sequential array transducer

38. Which of the following shortens the length of the pulse by decreasing the number of cycles in the pulse?
    a. Matching material
    b. Piezoelectric element
    c. Backing material
    d. Tungsten

39. Which of the following produces a pie-shaped image?
    a. Linear sequenced array
    b. Phased array
    c. Curved sequenced array
    d. Convex transducer

40. The portion of the transducer that comes in contact with the patient is the:
    a. Backing material
    b. Footprint
    c. Wire
    d. Damping material

41. What does heat sterilization do to an ultrasound transducer?
    a. Gives it better axial resolution
    b. Improves the lateral resolution of the transducer
    c. Kills all the bacteria and viruses
    d. Kills pathogens and destroys the transducer

42. Which of the following is defined as the minimum distance two reflectors can be, parallel to the beam, and still appear on the screen as two dots?
    a. Range resolution
    b. Angular resolution
    c. Contrast resolution
    d. Transverse resolution

43. Which of the following describes the result of destructive interference?
    a. The resulting wave is much larger than the original wave
    b. The resulting wave is a little larger than the original wave
    c. The resulting wave is smaller than the original wave
    d. Destructive interference does not occur with diagnostic imaging

44. To produce a transducer with a higher frequency one should:
    a. Use a thinner piezoelectric element
    b. Use a thicker piezoelectric element
    c. Use more damping
    d. Use less damping

45. Which of the following is not a characteristic of an unfocused single-element transducer?
    a. At the face of the transducer, the beam diameter is equal to the element diameter
    b. At a distance of one near zone length, the beam diameter is equal to one half of the diameter of the element
    c. At a distance of two near zone lengths, the beam diameter again equals the element diameter
    d. At the face of the transducer, the beam diameter is twice the size of the element thickness

46. Which of the following would be best utilized for imaging of deep structures in the abdomen?
    a. Linear phased array transducer
    b. Linear sequenced array transducer
    c. Curved sequenced array transducer
    d. Continuous-wave transducer

47. Which of the following is not a method of creating 3D images?
    a. Annular array transducer
    b. 2D array technology
    c. Freehand technique
    d. Mechanical technique

48. Which of the following best describes the frame rate?
    a. The frame rate is equal to the pulse repetition frequency multiplied by the lines per frame
    b. The frame rate is equal to the pulse repetition frequency divided by the lines per frame
    c. The frame rate is equal to the pulse repetition period divided by the lines per frame
    d. The frame rate is equal to the pulse repetition period multiplied by the lines per frame

49. Which of the following is represented as time, or the ability to display structures in real time?
    a. Temporal resolution
    b. Axial resolution
    c. Longitudinal resolution
    d. Contrast resolution

50. How are ultrasound transducers typically sterilized?
    a. Heating to the Curie temperature
    b. Cold-sterilization methods
    c. Autoclaving
    d. Alcohol emersion

SUGGESTED READINGS

Brant W. The Core Curriculum: Ultrasound. Philadelphia, PA: Lippincott Williams & Wilkins, 2001.
Bushberg JT, Seibert JA, Leidholdt EM, et al. The Essential Physics of Medical Imaging. 2nd Ed. Philadelphia, PA: Lippincott Williams & Wilkins, 2002.
Cosby K, Kendall J. Practical Guide to Emergency Ultrasound. Philadelphia, PA: Lippincott Williams & Wilkins, 2007.

Edelman SK. Understanding Ultrasound Physics. 3rd Ed. Woodlands, TX: ESP, Inc., 2005.

Hedrick WR, Hykes DL, Starchman DE. Ultrasound Physics and Instrumentation. 4th Ed. St. Louis, MO: Elsevier Mosby, 2005.

Kremkau FW. Diagnostic Ultrasound: Principles and Instruments. 7th Ed. St. Louis, MO: Saunders, 2006.

Miele FR. Ultrasound Physics & Instrumentation. 4th Ed. Forney, TX: Miele Enterprises LLC, 2006.

Sanders R, Winters T. Clinical Sonography: A Practical Guide. 4th Ed. Philadelphia, PA: Lippincott, Williams & Wilkins, 2007.

CHAPTER 3

Pulse–Echo Instrumentation

INTRODUCTION

This chapter discusses how sound is produced and what happens after the return echo is received by the transducer. Additionally, a description of the imaging artifacts that may occur as a result of sound transmission through soft tissue is offered.

KEY TERMS

13 μs rule—the rule that states that it takes 13 μs for sound to travel 1 cm in soft tissue

A-mode—amplitude mode; the height of the spike on the image is related to the strength (amplitude) of the echo generated by the reflector

ALARA—as low as reasonably achievable; the principle that states one should always use the lowest power and shortest scanning time possible to reduce potential exposure to the patient

amplification—the part of the receiver that increases or decreases the received echoes equally, regardless of depth

amplitude—the maximum or minimum deviation of an acoustic variable from the average value of that variable; the strength of the reflector

amplitude mode—*see key term A-mode*

analog-to-digital (A-to-D) converter—the part of the digital scan converter that converts the analog signals from the receiver to binary for processing by the computer

anechoic—without echoes, or black

apodization—the technique that varies the voltage to the individual elements to reduce grating lobes

artifacts—echoes on the screen that are not representative of actual anatomy, or reflectors in the body that are not displayed on the screen

B-mode—brightness mode; the brightness of the dots is proportional to the strength of the echo generated by reflector

beam former—the instrument that shapes and steers the beam on the transmit end

binary—the digital language of zeroes and ones

bistable—black-and-white image

bit—the smallest unit of memory in a digital device

brightness mode—*see key term B-mode*

byte—eight bits of memory

cathode ray tube (CRT)—display that uses an electron gun to produce a stream of electrons toward a phosphor-coated screen

coded excitation—a way of processing the pulse to improve contrast resolution and reduce speckle

comet tail—a type of reverberation artifact caused by small reflectors (i.e., surgical clips)

compensation—the function of the receiver that changes the brightness of the echo amplitudes to compensate for attenuation with depth

compression—the function of the receiver that decreases the range of signal amplitudes present with the machine's receiver; opposite of dynamic range

contrast resolution—the ability to differentiate one shade of gray from another

demodulation—the function of the receiver that makes the signal easier to process by performing rectification and smoothing

digital-to-analog (D-to-A) converter—part of the digital scan converter that converts the binary signals from computer memory to analog for display and storage

dynamic range—the series of echo amplitudes present within the signal

edge shadowing—refraction artifact caused by the curved surface of the reflector

electrical interference—arc-like bands that occur when the machine is too close to an unshielded electrical device

enhancement—an artifact caused by sound passing through an area of lower attenuation

field—one half of a frame on the display

fill-in interpolation—places pixels where there is no signal information based on adjacent scan lines

frame—one complete ultrasound image

frequency compounding—averages the frequencies across the image to improve contrast resolution and reduce speckle

fundamental frequency—the operating or resonating frequency emitted by the transducer

grating lobes—an artifact caused by extraneous sound not along primary beam path; occurs with arrays; reduced or eliminated by apodization, subdicing, and tissue harmonics

hyperechoic—displayed echoes that are relatively brighter than the surrounding tissue; may also be referred to as echogenic

hypoechoic—displayed echoes that are relatively darker than the surrounding tissue

liquid crystal display (LCD)—display that uses the twisting and untwisting of liquid crystals in front of a light source

M-mode—motion mode; used to display motion of the reflectors

master synchronizer—the timing component of the ultrasound machine that notes how long it takes for signals to return from reflectors (see key term range equation)

mirror image—an artifact caused by sound bouncing off of strong reflector and causing a structure to appear on both sides of the reflector

motion mode—see key term M-mode

multipath—an artifact caused by the beam bouncing off of several reflectors before returning to the transducer

nonlinear propagation—principle that pressure waves change in shape as they travel deeper, though in a disproportionate way

nonsinusoidal—waves that are not pure sine waves

output—output power; strength of sound entering the patient

overall gain—receiver function that increases or decreases all the echo amplitudes equally

PACS—Picture Archiving and Communication System; a type of display and storage device commonly used in ultrasound and other imaging modalities

pixel (picture element)—the smallest component of a 2D digital image

preprocessing—occurs in the A-to-D converter; the image must be live

postprocessing—occurs in the D-to-A converter; the image must be frozen

pulser—part of the beam former that controls the amount of energy in the pulse

range equation—equation used to calculate the distance to the reflector; in soft tissue, $d = 0.77t$ where "d" is the depth of the reflector and "t" represents the round-trip time of the pulse

read zoom—the type of magnification performed in the D-to-A converter (postprocessing) that magnifies the image by enlarging the pixels

receiver—the component of the machine that processes the signals coming back from the patient

rectification—the part of the receiver that inverts the negative voltages to positives

rejection—function of the receiver that is used to reduce image noise; sets a threshold below which the signal will not be displayed

reverberation—an artifact caused by the beam bouncing between two strong reflectors

ring-down—a type of reverberation artifact caused by air

scan converter—the part of the ultrasound machine that processes the signals from the receiver; consists of the A-to-D converter, computer memory, and D-to-A converter

scan line—created when one or more pulses of sound return from the tissue containing information related to the depth and amplitude of the reflectors

shadowing—an artifact caused by the failure of sound to pass through a strong attenuator

side lobes—an artifact caused by extraneous sound that is not found along the primary beam path; occurs with single-element transducers

smoothing—part of the demodulation component of the receiver; an "envelope" is wrapped around the signal to eliminate the "humps"

speckle reduction—algorithm used in signal processing to reduce the amount of acoustic speckle

subdicing—dividing the piezoelectric elements into very small pieces to reduce grating lobes

tissue harmonics—harmonic signal produced by the patient and is a multiple of the fundamental frequency; also referred to as native tissue harmonic imaging

TGC—time-gain compensation; *see key term* compensation

voxel (volume element)—the smallest component of a 3D image

write zoom—the type of magnification performed in the A-to-D converter (preprocessing) that magnifies the image by redrawing it before it is stored in memory

x-axis—the plane that is perpendicular to the beam path

y-axis—the plane that is parallel to the beam path

z-axis—the brightness, or amplitude, of the dots on the display

DISPLAY MODES

There are different modes used in ultrasound imaging for displaying the return echo information on the display (Table 3-1).

A-Mode

One of the original methods of displaying the return echo information was a display similar to an oscilloscope, where the depth was represented along the **x-axis** and the strength of the reflector was represented as a "spike" along the **y-axis**. A pulse of sound was sent out to create one **scan line** of information,

TABLE 3-1 Imaging modes.
Imaging Mode
A-mode
B-mode
M-mode

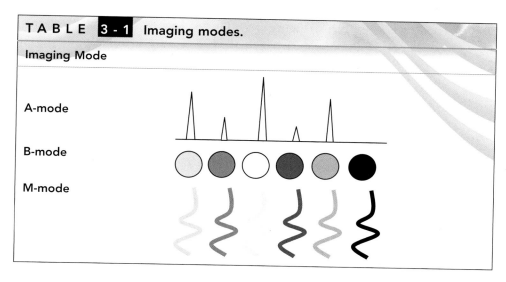

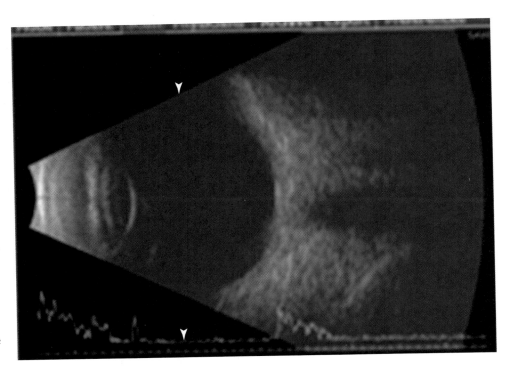

FIGURE 3-1 A-mode display superimposed over a B-mode image. Note that the amplitude (height) of the A-mode signal is proportional to the shade of gray on the B-mode image. Where the image is black the corresponding amplitude is very low (*arrows*). (Image courtesy of Wills Eye Hospital, Philadelphia, PA.)

which contained the depth and **amplitude** of the reflectors. No image was generated, only a set of spikes representing the amplitude of reflectors and their depth (Figure 3-1). This display method is called **amplitude mode** or **A-mode**, and it is still utilized in echocardiography and in dedicated ophthalmology/sonography units.

B-Mode

Brightness mode, or **B-mode** imaging, displays the return echoes as dots of varying brightnesses. The brightness of the dot represents the strength of the return echo (Figure 3-2). Modern equipment uses a white dot on a black background. The brighter the dot, the stronger the return echo. Very strong reflectors will be white or almost white (**hyperechoic**), weak reflectors will be a darker shade of gray (**hypoechoic**), and if there is no return echo information at all, then all that is seen at that location is black (**anechoic**) (Figure 3-3). That is to say, that a black space on the screen is absence of a return echo. This is why a full bladder appears anechoic. Simple fluids, such as water or urine, do not reflect much of the sound wave, so no dot is "painted" on the display in that area. The brightness of the dot representing the amplitude of the return echo corresponds to the height of the spike on the A-mode display. In fact, it is the same as the spike, but along the **z-axis** of the image (i.e., coming out of the display). Therefore, the amplitude of the B-mode image is displayed along the *z*-axis.

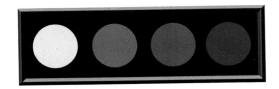

FIGURE 3-2 The different shades of gray.

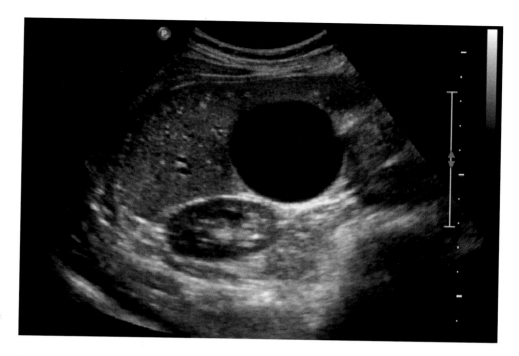

FIGURE 3-3 B-mode image of the upper abdomen.

The B-mode image is made up of many scan lines stacked next to each other. Each scan line is made up of one or more pulses of sound. In order for the machine to know where to place the dots on the screen, it has to know where the return echoes came from. In order to determine where the echo came from, the time it takes for the sound to reach the reflector and return must be known. This is summed up by the **range equation**, which states that the distance to the reflector (*d*, in millimeters) is equal to the propagation speed (*c*) multiplied by the round-trip time (*t*, in microseconds), or time to the reflector and back.

$$d = \frac{c \times t}{2}$$

To simplify the equation, because the ultrasound machine is programmed to always assume that the beam is traveling through soft tissue, the propagation speed of 1.54 mm/μs can be used to reveal an equation that assumes soft tissue: $d = 0.77t$. When answering questions about the depth of the reflector, verify that the information that is provided in the question is the round-trip time and not the one-way time. For example, if the time given is only *to the reflector*, you have to double it to make it the round-trip time. Important to know is the **13 μs rule**: it takes 13 μs (microseconds) for sound to travel to a depth of 1 cm and return (Table 3-2).

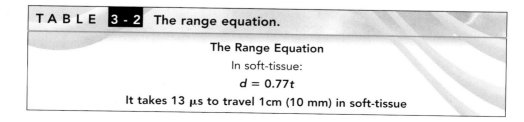

TABLE 3-2   The range equation.
The Range Equation
In soft-tissue:
$d = 0.77t$
It takes 13 μs to travel 1cm (10 mm) in soft-tissue

EXAMPLE 1: A sound wave travels 13 µs and impinges on a reflector. How far away is the reflector?

Note that in this example the round-trip time is not given, only the one-way time to the reflector. Therefore, the time given (13 µs) must be doubled and 26 µs plugged into the equation as follows: $d = 0.77(26 \text{ µs}) = 20$ mm. The distance to the reflector is 20 mm.

EXAMPLE 2: A reflector is 25 mm away from the transducer. How long does it take to get back to the transducer?

In this example, we are given the distance to the transducer and seeking the round-trip time. Rearrange the equation so that $t = d/0.77$.

$t = 25 \text{ mm}/0.77 = 32.46$ µs.

REMEMBER: t is the round-trip time. If the question asks "how long does it take for a pulse to get to the reflector?" the number provided should be divided in half.

M-Mode

With B-mode imaging, we are usually interested in the anatomy represented in the whole image. However, there are times when we are more concerned with the movement of the reflectors and not the anatomy. **M-mode**, or **motion mode**, is used in these instances when documentation of the movement of a reflector is needed, such as looking at the motion of a heart valve or myocardial wall thickness during systole and diastole. M-mode, is often used in obstetrics and in cardiac applications (Figure 3-4).

With M-mode imaging, the motion of the reflectors along a single scan line is analyzed. The M-mode tracing is one scan line represented over time with depth along the y-axis and time along the x-axis. This is sometimes referred to as "ice-pick" imaging because of the very narrow field-of-view. The M-mode image is one B-mode scan line represented over time (Figure 3-5).

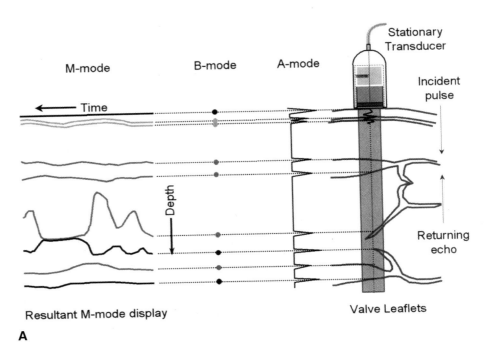

FIGURE 3-4 M-mode.
A. M-mode display of valve leaflets and corresponding appearance on A-mode and B-mode. (Image reprinted with permission from Bushberg J. The Essential Physics of Medical Imaging. 2nd Ed. Philadelphia, PA: Lippincott Williams & Wilkins, 2002:509.)

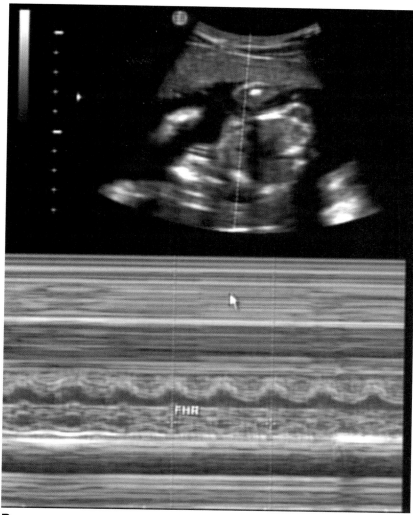

FIGURE 3-4 *(continued)* **B.** In this image, the M-mode tracing depicts the motion of the fetal heart.

B

TRANSMISSION OF ULTRASOUND

The ultrasound system is a complex piece of diagnostic equipment. Table 3-3 summarizes the components of an ultrasound machine.

Beam Former

The **beam former** controls the timing of the signals sent to the individual elements for steering and focusing of the beam. It is the job of the beam former to determine the sequence of the voltage pulses sent to the individual elements in an array transducer. These minute differences in timing steer and focus the beam (see Chapter 2). The beam former also controls **apodization**, which is used to decrease the risk of grating lobes. Apodization works by decreasing the strength of the voltage pulse sent to the outermost elements.

Pulser

The **pulser**, also referred to as the transmitter or pulse generator, controls the strength, or amplitude, of the electricity striking the elements, as well as the

FIGURE 3-5   One scan line.

TABLE 3-3 Parts of the ultrasound system and important points to remember.

Parts of the Ultrasound System	Important Points to Remember
Beam former	• Controls the timing of the elements to shape the beam for focusing • Controls the timing of the elements to steer the beam • Controls apodization
Pulser	• Part of the beam former • Generates the voltage that drives the transducer • Directly controls the amount of power entering the patient

Receiver	• Processes the return echo coming back from the patient
	  • Amplification: Increases or decreases all echoes equally
	  • Compensation: Adjusts brightness of echoes to correct for attenuation with depth
	  • Compression: Decreases the range of amplitudes present within the system (opposite of dynamic range)
	  • Demodulation: Makes signal easier for system to process. Includes rectification and smoothing
	  • Reject: Eliminates low-level echoes that do not contribute to useful information on the image

Scan converter	• A-to-D converter (preprocessing): Processes the signal before it is stored in memory. Converts analog signal to binary. Any function that has to be changed while the image is live is a preprocessing function • Digital memory: Uses computer memory (which uses binary language) to store the image information on an image matrix that corresponds to pixels on the display • D-to-A converter (postprocessing): Converts the binary back to analog form to get the signal ready for display and/or output to another medium (film, etc.). Settings that can be changed after the image has been frozen are postprocessing functions
Display	• CRT: Electron gun shoots stream of electrons to phosphor-coated screen. Beam is steered using magnetic fields • LCD: Flat-panel screen. Two polarized filters in front of a light source. Sandwiched between the filters are liquid crystals that twist/untwist with the application of electricity to determine if the backlighting gets through or not
Recording and storage	• Film: Not utilized much anymore. Paper may also used to be print images • PACS: Picture Archiving and Communication System. Uses a computer to store images. Can transmit images to remote locations. No films to lose • VHS: Magnetic tape storage • CD/DVD: Optical disk storage • MO disk: Magneto-optical disk storage

pulse repetition frequency and pulse repetition period. The strength of the sound wave entering the medium is directly proportional to the strength of the signal (voltage) impinging upon the elements. The stronger the output power used, the stronger the beam (i.e., higher the amplitude) of the sound entering the medium, and therefore the proportionally stronger the signal that returns from the reflectors in the medium (Figure 3-6). It is also important

FIGURE 3-6   Diagram depicting the direct relationship between amplitude voltage and amplitude signal strength. High amplitude voltage pulse equals high amplitude signal strength **(A)**, while low amplitude voltage pulse equals low amplitude signal strength **(B)**.

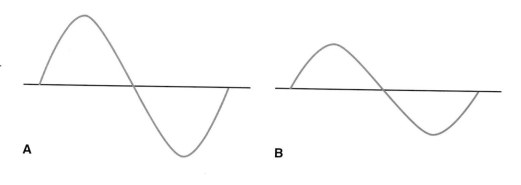

FIGURE 3-7   Diagram indicating that amplitude and frequency are independent of each other. **A.** Two waves of identical frequency and different amplitudes. **B.** Two waves having identical amplitudes but different frequencies.

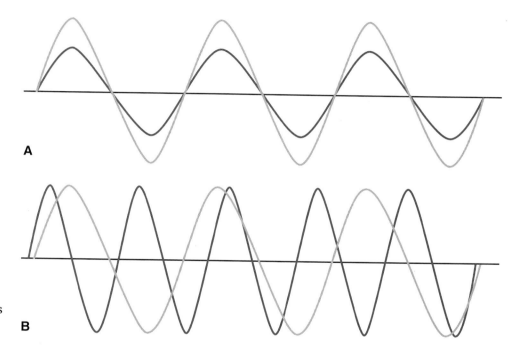

to note that frequency and amplitude are unrelated. Increasing or decreasing the strength of the pulse sent out of the transducer in no way changes the operating frequency of the transducer (Figure 3-7).

Power is known by several names (output, output gain, output power, acoustic power, etc.). Only the pulser controls the amount of power entering the patient. If the word "output" or "power" is used in a term (i.e., output gain), know that this is a pulser function. Keep in mind that the higher the output power, the stronger the return echo. Increased **output power** has a few beneficial side effects (1) higher amplitude return echoes for a better signal-to-noise ratio (i.e., less image noise) and (2) improved depth penetration. Increased output power is not without its disadvantage. Increasing the output power increases the exposure to the patient and therefore an increased risk of potential bioeffects. Therefore, the lowest power needed should always be used, following the principle of **ALARA** (as low as reasonably achievable), which states that the lowest power and shortest scanning time should be used to reduce the potential risk of bioeffects. If the image is too dark, the receiver gain should always be increased before output power.

Coded excitation is a more complicated way of driving the energy pulse. This technique sends a series of encoded pulses to form one scan line instead of the one-pulse-per-scan-line method. This technique allows for multiple focal zones, improved penetration, **speckle reduction**, B-flow imaging, and improved **contrast resolution**.

As discussed in Chapter 2, one side effect of damping is that pulsed-wave transducers have many frequencies in the beam (i.e., wide bandwidth). With **frequency compounding**, the soft tissue is imaged at various frequencies and averaged. The displayed image is the result of all of the frequencies and is another way to produce an image with improved contrast resolution and reduction in noise and speckle.

Master Synchronizer

The **master synchronizer** is the part of the machine responsible for controlling the timing of the echoes. This part of the machine tells the pulser to send out a pulse and pays attention to when the echoes come back to determine their range. The master synchronizer ensures that a new pulse is not sent out until the previous pulse has returned.

Tissue Harmonic Imaging

As stated in previous chapters, sound is a traveling pressure wave. As a pressure wave travels through tissue, its shape is deformed so that the high-pressure peak of the wave starts traveling faster than its low-pressure trough. The deeper the wave travels, the more deformed, or **nonsinusoidal**, it becomes. This is called **nonlinear propagation**. Because of the deformed wave, additional frequencies are generated in the tissue by the patient, called **tissue harmonics** (Table 3-4). At the surface no harmonics are generated; they are only generated as the beam travels deeper. The original frequency, called the **fundamental frequency**, is filtered out of the received beam and only the harmonic signal is processed. These harmonic signals are multiples of the fundamental frequency. It is the second harmonic, or two times the fundamental frequency, that is most often used. Therefore, if a 2-MHz beam is sent into the patient, the 4-MHz harmonic signal is what is displayed (Figure 3-8). This harmonic signal is very narrow, thereby offering excellent lateral resolution (Figure 3-9). As a result of harmonic signals being generated deep to the surface, most superficial **artifacts**, such as reverberation, are reduced or eliminated.

T A B L E 3 - 4 Important points concerning tissue harmonic imaging.
Tissue Harmonic Imaging
• Nonlinear propagation of sound
• Harmonic signals are produced by the patient, not the transducer
• Narrow beam—better lateral resolution
• Second harmonic is twice the transmitted (fundamental) frequency
• Elimination of near-field artifacts (noise, reverberation)
• Elimination of grating lobes
• Harmonic beam is weaker (lower amplitude than the fundamental) but travels only one way: from the patient to the transducer

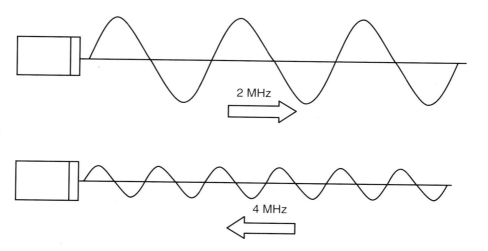

FIGURE 3-8 Diagram illustrating harmonic imaging. Fundamental frequency goes in at *x* frequency. Second harmonic signal is returned to the transducer at 2*x*, the fundamental frequency. For example, 2 MHz is fundamental transmitted into patient, and 4 MHz is the harmonic signal received from patient. The fundamental is filtered out and only the harmonic signal is used.

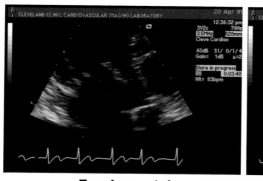
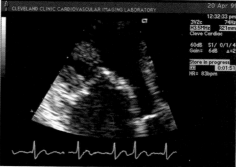

Fundamental   **Harmonic**

FIGURE 3-9 Harmonic imaging. In this patient with mitral stenosis, harmonic imaging **(right)** shows the endocardial definition and subvalvular apparatus with greater clarity than fundamental imaging **(left)**. (Image reprinted with permission from Topol EJ, Califf RM, et al. Textbook of Cardiovascular Medicine. 3rd Ed. Philadelphia, PA: Lippincott Williams & Wilkins, 2006.)

RECEPTION OF ULTRASOUND

Receiver

The return signal is processed first by the **receiver**, which may also be referred to as the signal processor. Sound returns to the transducer and strikes the piezoelectric element(s). Remember that sound is a pressure wave, so there is a mechanical force hitting the element, which causes electricity to be produced. Keep in mind that altering the following receiver functions does not change the amount of power entering the patient:

• **Amplification**, or **overall gain**, increases or decreases the strength of all of the returning echoes equally (Figure 3-10).

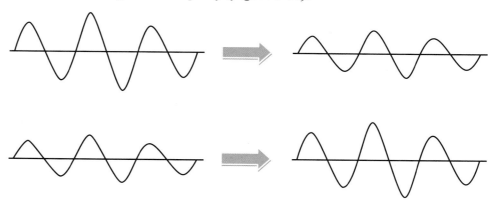

FIGURE 3-10 Amplification. All echo amplitudes increased or decreased equally, regardless of depth.

FIGURE 3-11 Depth gain compensation. **A.** Diagram showing the components of the time gain or depth gain compensation curve. **B.** Compensation "compensates" for the fact that attenuation occurs. The echoes farthest away from the transducer can be increased in brightness with the slide pot controls in order to achieve a more uniform level of brightness across the entire image. (Image reprinted with permission from Sanders R. Clinical Sonography: A Practical Guide. 4th Ed. Philadelphia, PA: Lippincott Williams & Wilkins, 2007:9.)

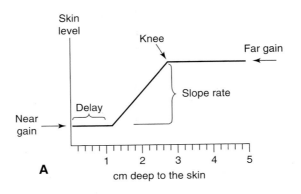

A

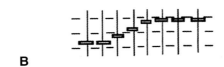

B

FIGURE 3-12 Compensation. Echo amplitudes increased in proportion to the attenuation that occurs (also known as TGC).

FIGURE 3-13 Compression. Compression is needed to decrease the difference between the largest and smallest amplitudes within the signal (the dynamic range). **A.** Signal before compression is applied. Notice the large difference between the largest signal amplitude and the smallest. **B.** Signal after compression is applied. Compression decreases the differences between the largest and smallest amplitudes.

- **Compensation**, also referred to as **TGC** or depth-gain compensation (DGC) adjusts for the strength of echoes in a different way. As the beam travels, the signal strength decreases due to attenuation. Therefore, the echoes farther away from the transducer will be weaker than the ones that are closer. Compensation "compensates" for the fact that attenuation occurs, and the farther-away or distant echoes are increased in brightness to achieve a uniform level of brightness on the image (Figures 3-11 and 3-12).
- **Compression** is needed to decrease the difference between the largest and smallest amplitudes within the signal (the **dynamic range**) (Figure 3-13).
- **Demodulation** processes the signal to make it easier for the machine to handle. The two components of demodulation are rectification and smoothing. **Rectification** turns negative voltages into positive voltages,

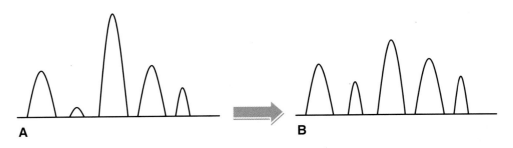

A   B

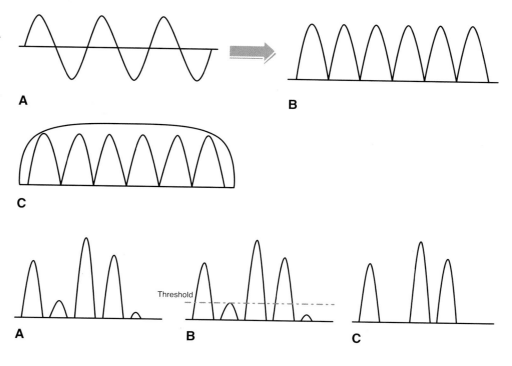

FIGURE 3-14 Demodulation. Demodulation processes the signal to make it easier for the machine to handle. Two components: **(A)** rectification turns negative voltages into positive voltages **(B)**, and smoothing **(C)** wraps an envelope around the signal to make it less "bumpy."

FIGURE 3-15 Rejection. Rejection discards signal amplitudes below a certain threshold to reduce image noise. **A.** Signal before rejection is applied. **B.** The threshold eliminates "noise" by removing signals below a certain set point. **C.** Signal result.

while **smoothing** wraps an envelope around the signal to make it less "bumpy" (Figure 3-14).

- **Rejection** discards signal amplitudes below a certain threshold to reduce image noise (Figure 3-15).

Scan Converter

The **scan converter** is the part of the machine that makes gray-scale imaging possible and is responsible for storage of the image data. The initial scan converters were all analog. Analog means infinite, and these scan converters could store a large range of signal amplitudes allowing for many shades of gray. An often-used example of an analog device is the dimmer switch. Present-day scan converters are digital devices. Digital means finite, in that there are far less choices available. For example, whereas the dimmer switch lets you adjust an infinitely variable light setting, the on–off switch is a "digital" device, in that you have discrete, finite choices (on or off, with nothing in between). Digital devices such as computers use the binary system, which utilizes only zeroes and ones instead of the numbers zero through nine. Computers only communicate and process signals in binary, so any signal coming into the computer has to be converted into zeroes and ones. In ultrasound machines, signals are represented by black-and-white dots, or echoes; zero (0) represents "off," or a black echo, while one (1) represents "on," or a white echo. Before scan converters made gray-scale imaging possible, images were purely black and white, or **bistable**.

Signals travel from the receiver to the scan converter, which consists of the **analog-to-digital (A-to-D) converter**, computer memory, and the **digital-to-analog (D-to-A) converter**. **Preprocessing** of the signal occurs in the A-to-D converter, where incoming signals are assigned shades of gray based on their amplitudes. At this point the image is still "live." Any changes to the image that need to be made while the image is live occur in the A-to-D converter and therefore are preprocessing functions.

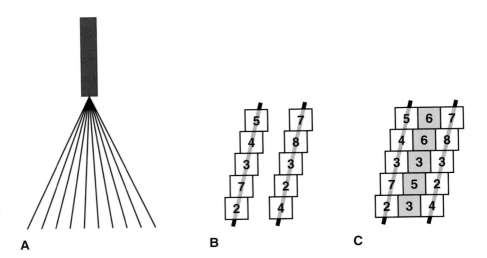

A **B** **C**

There are occasions where gaps exist between the scan lines, such as the diverging scan lines of sector scans. In these cases, the machine guesses what pixel should be placed there based on the surrounding shades of gray, a process called **fill-in interpolation** (Figure 3-16). After the signal is converted to a digital form, it can be processed by the computer. The computer is where the image is stored so it can be displayed.

Computers use the **binary system**, where the image information is made up of zeroes and ones (Table 3-5). A **bit** is the smallest amount of computer memory possible. Eight bits = 1 **byte**. The number of bits in memory determines the number of shades of gray possible. With only one bit there are only two shades available: black and white (or bistable). The formula to determine the number of shades of gray is 2^n, where n is the number of bits. Two bits of memory = 4 shades of gray (2^2). Eight bits of memory = 256 shades of gray (2^8).

The digital computer has a location in its memory for every **pixel** on the display. A pixel is short for picture element, the smallest part of any picture. The more pixels on a display, the better the spatial resolution of the display. Therefore, an image matrix of 512×512 pixels is better than 256×256 pixels. In general, it is better to have more pixels than it is to have more shades of gray (Figure 3-17). For 3D imaging, the term used is **voxel**, which is short for volume element. Table 3-6 sums up computer terminology.

Once the signal is stored in memory, it is sent to the D-to-A converter. This is a component of the **postprocessing** part of the digital scan converter. In the D-to-A converter, the signal is converted back to analog form so it can be displayed and sent to **PACS**, film, video, and so on. Although the image is frozen at this point, on many machines there are certain image settings that can be changed, such as the displayed range of shades of gray in the image.

There are two different ways of magnifying the ultrasound image: **write zoom** and **read zoom** (Figure 3-18). Write zoom, a preprocessing function, enlarges the image by redrawing it. As the image has not been stored in memory yet, it is therefore possible to enlarge the image while maintaining the pixel density. This offers a high-quality zoomed image. Write zoom is a preprocessing function, so it occurs in the A-to-D converter and therefore the image must be live. Read zoom, a postprocessing function, enlarges the image by magnifying the pixels. The image has already been stored in

TABLE 3-5　Binary conversion.

To convert TO binary:

Converting to binary is not difficult: just remember the number ONE.

- Create a table of columns
- Starting with the **right-hand** column, write the number one
- Populate the remaining columns (working right to left) by doubling the number

16	8	4	2	1

- How far to the left do you need to go? Depends on what you want to convert. For example, to convert the number 30 to binary, you go no higher than the number 30. Try it: Fill out the grid below by doubling, starting with the number one:

32	16	8	4	2	1

- Look at the leftmost column—notice it is a 32. That is higher than 30, so ignore it or do not write it. You do not need it. The highest column we need is 16. How many times does 16 go into 32? The answer can *only* be a <u>zero</u> or a <u>one</u>. Sixteen goes into 30 one time, so we put a one under the "16" column, as follows:

16	8	4	2	1
1				

- You have to subtract 16 from the original 30 now, because you just used it up
  - 30 − 16 = 14. Move down the column. How many times does 8 go into 14? Once, so add the "1" under the "8"

16	8	4	2	1
1	1			

- Now subtract 8 from 14
  - 14 − 8 = 6. How many times does 4 go into 6? Once, so add it under the "4"

16	8	4	2	1
1	1	1		

  - 6 − 4 = 2. How many times does 2 go into 2? Once, so add it under the "2"

16	8	4	2	1
1	1	1	1	

  - 2 − 2 = 0. How many times does 1 go into 0? None, so add a 0 under the "1"

16	8	4	2	1
1	1	1	1	0

- There you have it! The binary of 30 is **11110**

To convert FROM binary:

To convert from binary, look at how many digits there are in the number. For example, 11110 has five digits. Draw a grid, with as many columns as there are digits.

16	8	4	2	1

- Five digits, five columns. Now, populate the columns with the binary number

16	8	4	2	1
1	1	1	1	0

- All of the columns that have a "1" in it, add those up.
- 16 + 8 + 4 + 2 = <u>30</u>

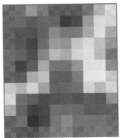
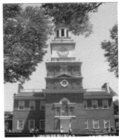
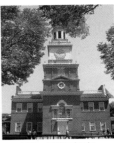

10 x 12 pixels   128 x 155 pixels   413 x 500 pixels

FIGURE 3-17 Pixels. In general, it is better to have more pixels than it is to have more shades of gray. The more pixels on a display, the better the spatial resolution of that display. (Image courtesy of Wikimedia Commons.)

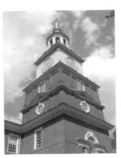
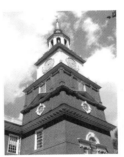
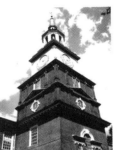
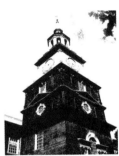

256 shades of gray   16 shades of gray   4 shades of gray   2 shades of gray (bistable)

TABLE 3-6 Computer terminology and description.

Computer Terminology	Description
Binary	Computer language of zeroes and ones
Bit	Binary digit. The smallest amount of computer memory
Byte	Eight bits of memory
Pixel	A picture element. The smallest unit of a 2D image
Voxel	A volume element. The smallest unit of a 3D image
Image matrix	Storage in memory corresponding to each pixel on the display

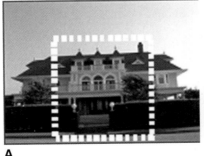
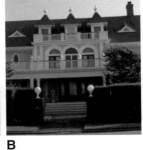
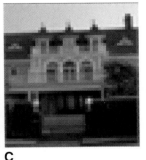

A   B   C

FIGURE 3-18 Write zoom verses read zoom. The original image **(A)** in this diagram is being analyzed. Write zoom is a preprocessing function that enlarges the image by redrawing it **(B)**. This offers a high-quality zoomed image. Read zoom, a postprocessing function, enlarges the image by making the pixels bigger **(C)**. This type of zoom offers a courser, less optimal type of zoom.

TABLE 3-7 Write and read zoom comparison.	
Write Zoom	**Read Zoom**
Preprocessing function	Postprocessing function
A-to-D converter	D-to-A converter
Image must be live	Image may be frozen or live
Higher-quality zoom	Lower-quality zoom
Write zoom is the "write" way to do it!	

memory, so it is not possible to maintain the pixel density. This type of zoom offers a courser, less optimal type of zoom. With read zoom, the image may be frozen or live. To remember which is which, remember: Write zoom is the "write" way to do it (Table 3-7).

Display

There are two displays used as ultrasound monitors: **cathode ray tubes (CRTs)** or **liquid crystal displays (LCDs)** (Figures 3-19 and 3-20). The CRT is like a television. It works by using an electron gun to send a stream of electrons toward a phosphor-coated screen. The beam is steered via the use of magnetic deflector coils. The image is interlaced; that is, a single 525-line **frame** (image) is made up of two **fields**, even and odd. The odd field (line 1, 3, 5, . . . , 525) is placed on the screen first with the electron beam, and then the even field (2, 4, 6, . . . , 524). It takes 1/60th of a second to produce each field. Therefore, since two fields make one frame, it takes 1/30th of a second to display one frame, or one ultrasound image, on a CRT. The conventional CRT can therefore display 30 frames per second (30 fps, or 30 Hz). The LCD, or flat-panel display, works with a light source positioned behind two polarized filters with liquid crystals sandwiched between them. The twisting or untwisting of the crystals determines if light shines through to the face of the display.

Recording and Storage Devices

PACS is the most recent display and storage medium (Figures 3-21 and 3-22). Other storage devices include all of the following: film, video recording,

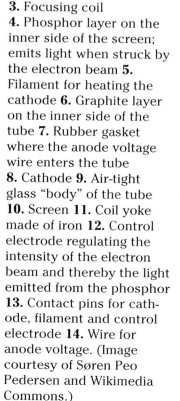

FIGURE 3-19   Diagram of a cathode ray tube. **1.** Deflection coils **2.** Electron beam **3.** Focusing coil **4.** Phosphor layer on the inner side of the screen; emits light when struck by the electron beam **5.** Filament for heating the cathode **6.** Graphite layer on the inner side of the tube **7.** Rubber gasket where the anode voltage wire enters the tube **8.** Cathode **9.** Air-tight glass "body" of the tube **10.** Screen **11.** Coil yoke made of iron **12.** Control electrode regulating the intensity of the electron beam and thereby the light emitted from the phosphor **13.** Contact pins for cathode, filament and control electrode **14.** Wire for anode voltage. (Image courtesy of Søren Peo Pedersen and Wikimedia Commons.)

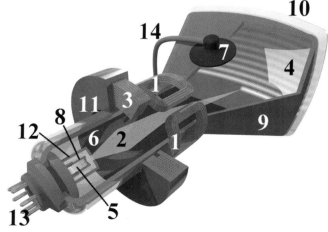

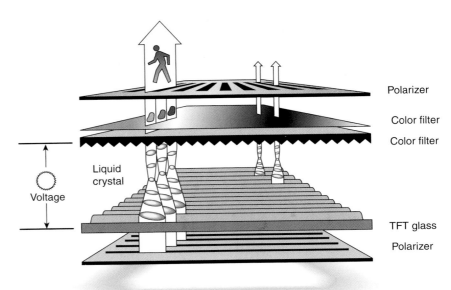

FIGURE 3-20 Diagram of an LCD. (Image courtesy of Wikimedia Commons.)

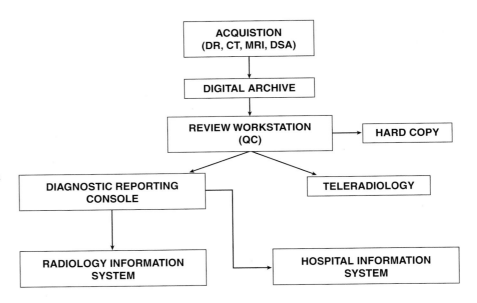

FIGURE 3-21 Diagram of a PACS system. (Image reprinted with permission from Daffner, RH. Clinical Radiology: The Essentials. 3rd Ed. Philadelphia, PA: Lippincott Williams & Wilkins, 2007.)

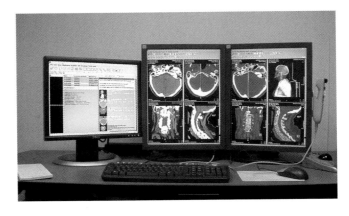

FIGURE 3-22 Photograph of a PACS workstation. (Image reprinted with permission from Daffner, RH. Clinical Radiology: The Essentials. 3rd Ed. Philadelphia, PA: Lippincott Williams & Wilkins, 2007.)

such as VHS, which uses a magnetic tape, CD/DVD, which are optical storage devices, and magneto-optical (MO) storage. Images can also be sent to paper or thermal printers. PACS systems use a RAID (redundant array of independent disks) to store large quantities of data.

IMAGING ARTIFACTS

Artifacts are echoes on the screen that are not representative of actual anatomic features or occur when there are anatomic structures in the body that are not displayed on the screen (Table 3-8). Artifacts may also occur as a result of electrical interference or a problem with the ultrasound machine.

Artifacts result from assumptions that the ultrasound machine makes. These include:

- Sound beams travel in a straight line and go directly from the transducer and back.
- The only propagation speed in the body is 1540 m/s.

TABLE 3-8 Imaging artifacts.

Imaging Artifacts	Description
Reverberation	Closely spaced parallel echoes of decreasing brightness deep to two parallel specular reflectors
Mirror image	Artifact caused by sound reflecting off of strong specular reflector and displaying an object on both sides of the reflector
Multipath	Beam reflects off of objects in body and makes two or more changes in direction before returning back to transducer
Edge shadowing	Refraction artifact caused by sound refracting off of curved surface. Eliminated/reduced by spatial compounding
Side lobes/Grating lobes	Extraneous energy not along path of main beam causes erroneous reflections
Propagation speed errors	If the actual propagation speed of the tissue is greater than or less than 1540 m/s, the machine places the reflector at the wrong location on the display. Remember: The machine is using $d = 0.77t$
Shadowing	Potentially useful artifact occurs when sound traverses a highly attenuating structure. Helps to identify stones
Enhancement	Useful artifact occurs when sound travels through a weakly attenuating structure. Appears as an area of increased brightness distal to weak reflectors
Slice thickness artifact (also known as elevational plane artifact)	Artifact that occurs as a result of the beam not being razor thin. Unintended echoes may appear in the image as the beam slices through structures adjacent to intended reflectors
Electric interference	Disturbance on display that appears as "arc-like" moving bands caused by the ultrasound machine being placed too close to unshielded electrical equipment

- Any reflection that comes back to the transducer must have been along the path of the beam.
- The slice thickness plane is razor thin.

A common artifact is **reverberation**, which occurs when the sound bounces back and forth between two close-together strong specular reflectors (Figure 3-23). This produces a "step-ladder"-like appearance of parallel echoes that are equally spaced and decrease in brightness (amplitude) with depth. Two subtypes of reverberation include **comet tail** (caused by small structures like surgical clips) (Figure 3-24) and **ring-down** (usually caused by small air bubbles) (Figure 3-25).

Mirror image artifact occurs when the sound is aimed toward a large specular reflector that acts like a mirror and directs some of the sound in a direction

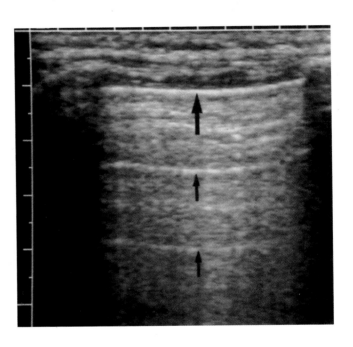

FIGURE 3-23
Reverberation artifact. Intercostal linear array image of the normal lung surface shows intense reflections at the soft tissue–air interface *(large arrow)* that reflects back and forth between the transducer surface and the interface to produce a series of reverberation bands *(small arrows)* deeper in the image. (Image reprinted with permission from Brant W. Ultrasound. Philadelphia, PA: Lippincott Williams & Wilkins, 2001:15.)

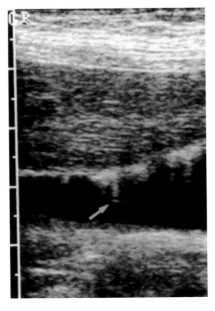

FIGURE 3-24 Comet tail artifact. Image of the gallbladder shows a series of bright tapering echoes *(arrow)* extending from its walls. This is a sonographic finding that is commonly associated with cholesterol crystal accumulation within the gallbladder wall, a condition known as adenomyomatosis. (Image reprinted with permission from Brant W. Ultrasound. Philadelphia, PA: Lippincott Williams & Wilkins, 2001:15.)

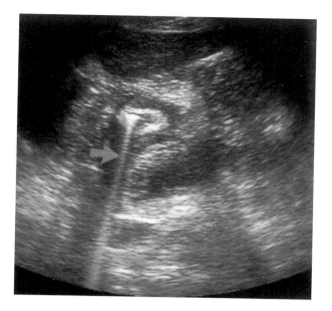

FIGURE 3-25 Ring-down artifact. Longitudinal image of the gastric antrum shows a prominent ring-down artifact *(arrow)* caused by air bubbles in the stomach. (Image reprinted with permission from Brant W. Ultrasound. Philadelphia, PA: Lippincott Williams & Wilkins, 2001:16.)

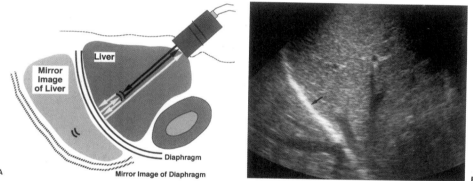

FIGURE 3-26 Mirror image artifact. **A.** Near-complete reflection of the sound beam from the surface of the air-filled lung above the diaphragm causes a reflection of the beam back and forth with the liver before finally returning to the transducer. The prolonged time-of-flight of these delayed echoes results in an artifactual display of the liver parenchyma above the diaphragm. **B.** Mirror image artifact duplicates the hepatic veins and liver above the diaphragm *(arrow)*. (Image reprinted with permission from Brant W. Ultrasound. Philadelphia, PA: Lippincott Williams & Wilkins, 2001:18.)

other than back to the transducer. This causes the reflector to appear equally spaced apart from either side of the strong reflector. This artifact is commonly seen near the diaphragm and pleura. Note that the duplicate object always appears deeper than the actual structure being duplicated (Figure 3-26).

Multipath artifact occurs when the beam strikes an interface and veers off in another direction. It changes direction a few times before returning to the transducer. This causes reflectors to be placed in the wrong location on the image.

Refraction causes artifacts as the beam is directed away from the path in which it was originally intended to go. One refraction artifact is **edge shadowing**, which is seen when sound strikes a curved reflector like the transverse gallbladder or carotid artery (Figure 3-27). Spatial compounding eliminates edge shadowing because the beam hits the structure at different angles.

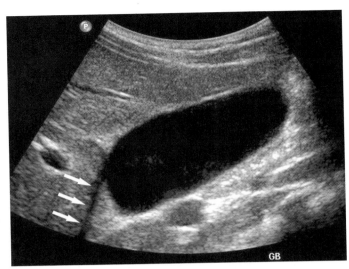

FIGURE 3-27 Edge shadow. Edge shadow *(arrows)* arising from the edge of the gallbladder. (Image reprinted with permission from Sanders R. Clinical Sonography: A Practical Guide. 4th Ed. Philadelphia, PA: Lippincott Williams & Wilkins, 2007:630.)

It is expected that sound energy travels along the main axis of the beam. If there is extraneous sound energy not along the main axis, the possibility exists that this sound will cause reflections back to the transducer. As the machine assumes that all reflectors lie along the path of the beam, the artifacts produced are called **side lobes** or **grating lobes** (Figures 3-28 and 3-29). Side lobes occur with all transducers and grating lobes occur with linear transducers. Tissue harmonics, apodization, and **subdicing** (slicing the crystals into even smaller sections) have largely reduced or eliminated grating lobes.

The machine assumes that the sound travels through all tissues at 1540 m/s, but this is not what actually happens. In the body, the different tissues actually have different propagation speeds, but the machine uses 1540 m/s regardless of which type of tissue the beam is traveling. If the actual propagation speed through which the sound is traveling is less than 1540 m/s, reflectors will be displayed on the screen too far away. Likewise, if the actual

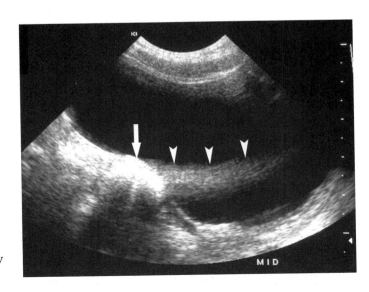

FIGURE 3-28 Sidelobe artifact. Longitudinal view of the urinary bladder showing sidelobe artifact *(arrowheads)* arising from bowel gas *(arrow)* extending well into the bladder. (Image reprinted with permission from Sanders R. Clinical Sonography: A Practical Guide. 4th Ed. Philadelphia, PA: Lippincott Williams & Wilkins, 2007:636. Courtesy of Piotr Niznik.)

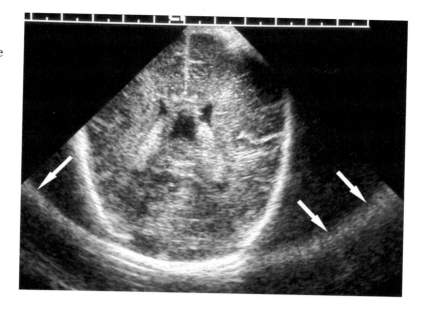

FIGURE 3-29 Grating lobe artifact. Coronal view of the neonatal brain using a phased array transducer. A grating lobe artifact *(arrows)* is seen arising from the occipital bone and extending laterally to the edge of the display. (Image reprinted with permission from Sanders R. Clinical Sonography: A Practical Guide. 4th Ed. Philadelphia, PA: Lippincott Williams & Wilkins, 2007:637.)

propagation speed of the tissue is greater than 1540 m/s, reflectors will be displayed too close.

Two particularly useful artifacts are **shadowing** and **enhancement**. Shadowing occurs when the sound travels through an area of higher attenuation (such as a rib or other calcified/bony structure) compared with the surrounding tissue (Figure 3-30). This artifact is useful because it helps with the identification of stones. Enhancement occurs from traveling through areas of lower attenuation, such as fluid (Figure 3-31). Because less of the sound is attenuated when traveling through this region (e.g., a cyst), there is more signal strength distal to the object. This makes the tissue deep to the weak attenuator appear brighter.

The ultrasound beam is not razor thin; it has a definite thickness in what is called the slice thickness, or elevational plane. Any reflectors appearing in this plane will appear in the image, even if you were looking at something else. An often-seen example of this is scanning through an ovarian cyst and seeing what appears to be echoes within it. After the transducer is turned 90°, the echoes disappear, indicating they are not really within the cyst.

FIGURE 3-30 Shadowing from a gallstone. This large gallstone within the gallbladder creates a dark shadow. (Image reprinted with permission from Cosby KS. Practical Guide to Emergency Ultrasound. Philadelphia, PA: Lippincott Williams & Wilkins, 2005.)

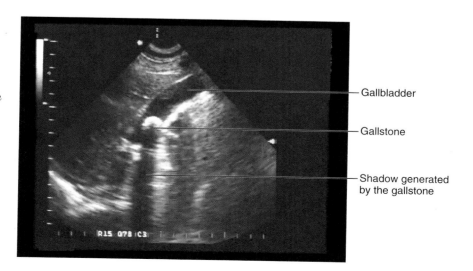

FIGURE 3-31
Enhancement. Longitudinal view of the spleen showing acoustic enhancement (*between arrows*) posterior to a splenic cyst (Cy). (Image reprinted with permission from Sanders R. Clinical Sonography: A Practical Guide. 4th Ed. Philadelphia, PA: Lippincott Williams & Wilkins, 2007:630.)

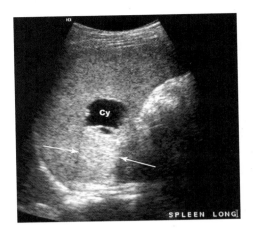

Slice thickness artifact occurs because the beam scanned through both the cyst and the soft tissue adjacent to the cyst, causing both to appear on the image. The solution to slice thickness artifact is better focusing in the elevational plane, such as with 1.5D transducers (see Chapter 2).

The presence of electrical equipment near the ultrasound machine (e.g., unshielded ventilators) may cause an artifact related to **electrical interference**. This causes arc-like bands that move across the screen as long as the machine is in the proximity of the unshielded equipment.

REVIEW QUESTIONS

1. The output gain of the pulser determines the _____ of the acoustic pulse.
   a. Frequency
   b. Intensity
   c. Duration
   d. Pulse repetition period

2. What is the receiver function that adjusts the image because of the darker appearance of reflectors in the far field as a result of attenuation?
   a. Compression
   b. Compensation
   c. Confirmation
   d. Condensation

3. Which of the following tasks is incorporated in the process of demodulation?
   a. Rejection
   b. Rectification
   c. Amplification
   d. Receiving

4. What is the smallest element in a digital picture called?
   a. The bit
   b. The pixel
   c. The byte
   d. The fractal

5. What is the name for the smallest amount of digital storage?
   a. The bit
   b. The pixel
   c. The byte
   d. The fractal

6. What receiver function converts the negative portion of the signal to positive?
   a. Compression
   b. Condensation
   c. Rectification
   d. Amplification

7. A video display that is limited to only black and white, with no other shades of gray, is called _____.
   a. Binary
   b. Monochrome
   c. Bistable
   d. Unichrome

8. In a standard cathode ray tube used to display ultrasound images, what are the charged particles that are emitted from a "gun" from the rear of the tube?
   a. Neutrons
   b. Photons
   c. Positrons
   d. Electrons

9. How does a cathode ray tube steer the charged particles emitted by the electron so that they sweep across the front screen?
   a. Phasing
   b. Mechanical steering
   c. Using a magnetic field
   d. Reflecting off of a mirror

10. Which of the following is a true statement?
    a. There are two frames in a field
    b. There are two fields in a frame
    c. One frame takes 1/60th of a second
    d. It takes 1/60th of a second to draw two fields

11. With 6 bits, what is the largest number of different shades of gray that can be stored?
    a. 64
    b. 8
    c. 256
    d. 16

12. In B-mode imaging, the stronger the return echo,
    a. The darker the dot on the display
    b. The brighter the dot on the display
    c. The worse the temporal resolution
    d. The weaker the transmit power

13. What happens to a digital image when the pixel density is increased?
    a. There is more spatial detail
    b. There is less spatial detail
    c. The temporal resolution increases
    d. There are more shades of gray

14. You are using a transducer that produces a beam with a very wide elevational plane. Which of the following problems are you most likely to encounter as a result?
    a. Slice thickness artifact
    b. Increased reverberation
    c. Increased side lobes
    d. Increased electrical interference

15. The "useful" artifact that one might see behind a weakly attenuating structure is:
    a. Shadowing
    b. Enhancement
    c. Reflection
    d. Refraction

16. When you adjust the output power control, you affect the following system component:
    a. Pulser
    b. Memory
    c. Scan converter
    d. Receiver

17. The part of the receiver that reduces low-level system noise is the:
    a. Demodulation
    b. Compensation
    c. Amplification
    d. Rejection

18. What receiver function is responsible for decreasing the difference between the largest and smallest received signal amplitudes?
    a. Amplification
    b. Compensation
    c. Compression
    d. Rejection

19. Sound bouncing off of a strong reflector and producing an image on the wrong location on the display is:
    a. Range ambiguity
    b. Mirror image artifact
    c. Slice thickness artifact
    d. Enhancement

20. What must be known in order to calculate distance to a reflector?
    a. Attenuation, speed, density
    b. Attenuation, impedance
    c. Density, speed
    d. Travel time, speed

21. Contrast resolution is:
    a. The ability to see differences in shades of gray
    b. The ability to display moving structures in real time
    c. The ability to identify two reflectors parallel to the beam
    d. The ability to identify two reflectors perpendicular to the beam

22. Which of the following occurs in the D-to-A converter?
    a. Preprocessing
    b. Postprocessing
    c. Conversion to binary
    d. Write zoom

23. In which mode is the strength of the reflector represented by the brightness of the dot?
    a. A-mode
    b. B-mode
    c. A and B
    d. None of the above

24. Which mode is interested in the movement of the reflectors along one scan line?
    a. A-mode
    b. B-mode
    c. M-mode
    d. C-mode

25. In M-mode imaging, what is along the x-axis?
    a. Depth
    b. Amplitude
    c. Intensity
    d. Time

26. The harmonic signal
    a. Is produced by the transducer
    b. Is produced by the patient
    c. Is of a stronger amplitude than the fundamental
    d. Has worse lateral resolution than the fundamental

27. When imaging in tissue harmonic imaging,
    a. The fundamental frequency is filtered out
    b. The fundamental beam's frequency is increased
    c. The harmonic signal is filtered out
    d. There are more artifacts

28. A sound wave travels 26 μs to a reflector. How far away is the reflector, assuming the medium is soft tissue?
    a. 0.5 cm
    b. 1.0 cm
    c. 2.0 cm
    d. 4.0 cm

29. A reflector is 20 mm away from the transducer. How long does it take for sound to get back to the transducer?
    a. 13 μs
    b. 20 μs
    c. 26 μs
    d. 39 μs

30. Which of the following is a technique used to reduce the presence of grating lobes?
    a. Apodization
    b. Tissue harmonics
    c. Subdicing
    d. All of the above

31. The strength of the voltages sent to each element is determined by the:
    a. Beam former
    b. Receiver
    c. Scan converter
    d. Display

32. An advantage of coded excitation is improved
    a. Azimuthal resolution
    b. Temporal resolution
    c. Signal-to-noise ratio
    d. Lateral resolution

33. If the far field of the image is too dark, it is recommended that you
    a. Do not press as hard on the patient
    b. Increase the receiver gain
    c. Increase the output gain
    d. Increase scanning time

34. Read zoom is a function of the:
    a. D-to-A converter
    b. A-to-D converter
    c. Preprocessing
    d. Pulser

35. Which type of zoom offers a high-quality zoom but must be selected while the image is live?
    a. Postprocessing zoom
    b. Read zoom
    c. Write zoom
    d. None of the above

36. As the sound beam travels it is attenuated. This explains the need to have which receiver function?
    a. Compression
    b. Demodulation
    c. Amplification
    d. Compensation

37. The smallest component of a 3D image is the:
    a. Bit
    b. Byte
    c. Voxel
    d. Pixel

38. The technique that uses made-up pixel information to replace areas between the scan lines where there is no actual signal information is:
    a. Compression
    b. Fill-in interpolation
    c. Tissue harmonics
    d. Frequency compounding

39. Which of the following is a storage medium that uses a magnetic tape?
    a. Film
    b. Thermal printer
    c. VHS
    d. CD

40. An artifact that occurs when a sound beam bounces back and forth between two strong reflectors, creating a "step-ladder"-like appearance is:
    a. Reverberation
    b. Side lobes

c. Multipath
d. Edge shadowing

41. Additional reflectors on the screen (with an array transducer) that are from extraneous sound waves off the primary axis of the beam are:
    a. Ring-down artifacts
    b. Edge shadows
    c. Side lobes
    d. Grating lobes

42. Sound travels through a large quantity of muscle tissue. The reflector will be displayed
    a. Too close to the transducer
    b. Too far away from the transducer
    c. In the correct location
    d. Sound does not travel through muscle tissue.

43. A shadow occurs when sound
    a. Travels through an area of decreased attenuation
    b. Travels through an area of increased attenuation
    c. Reflects off a weak attenuator
    d. Travels through a cystic structure

44. The echo information is taken from the memory and converted so it can be shown on the display in the:
    a. Beam former
    b. Receiver
    c. A-to-D converter
    d. D-to-A converter

45. Which older mode is still used today in ophthalmology?
    a. A-mode
    b. B-mode
    c. M-mode
    d. C-mode

46. Which part of the US machine does not affect the amount of energy entering the patient?
    a. Receiver
    b. Pulser
    c. Transmitter
    d. Beam former

47. An image with one bit of memory has how many shades of gray?
    a. None
    b. One
    c. Two
    d. Four

48. The part of the machine responsible for timing the reception of the pulses to determine their location is the:
    a. Beam former
    b. Scan converter
    c. Master synchronizer
    d. Display

49. A technique that averages out the frequencies used to make the image to improve contrast resolution and reduce speckle is:
    a. Spatial compounding
    b. Frequency compounding
    c. Coded excitation
    d. Tissue harmonics

50. Artifacts related to propagation speed occur because
    a. The machine can measure the propagation speed of the tissue
    b. The beam bounces off of strong reflectors
    c. The beam travels in a straight line
    d. The machine assumes 1540 m/s for all tissue

SUGGESTED READINGS

Feldman MK, Katyal S, Blackwood MS. US artifacts. Radiographics. 2009;29: 1179–1189.

Hedrick WR, Hykes DL, Starchman DE. Ultrasound Physics and Instrumentation. 4th Ed. St. Louis, MO: Elsevier Mosby, 2005.

Hughes S. Sonography Principles and Instrumentation. Plano, TX: Society of Diagnostic Medical Sonographers, 2009.

Kremkau FW. Diagnostic Ultrasound: Principles and Instruments. 7th Ed. St. Louis, MO: Saunders, 2006.

Miele FR. Ultrasound Physics & Instrumentation. 4th Ed. Forney, TX: Miele Enterprises LLC, 2006.

Tranquart F, Grenier N, Eder V, et al. Clinical use of ultrasound tissue harmonic imaging. Ultrasound in Medicine and Biology. 1999;25(6):889–894.

CHAPTER 4

Hemodynamics and Doppler Principles

OUTLINE

INTRODUCTION

This chapter is divided into two parts. The first part will cover hemodynamics, the science of how and why blood flows through the blood vessels of the body. Normal arterial and venous flow will be examined, as well as what happens when there is a stenosis. The second part of the chapter will discuss Doppler, review the Doppler equation, spectral, color, and power Doppler, as well as the artifacts that are associated with Doppler examinations.

KEY TERMS

aliasing—the wraparound of the spectral or color Doppler display that occurs when the frequency shift exceeds the Nyquist limit; only occurs with pulsed-wave Doppler

angle correct—the tool used to inform the machine what the flow angle is so that velocities can be accurately calculated

autocorrelation—the color Doppler processing technique that assesses pixels as stationary or in motion

BART—acronym used in echocardiography describing color Doppler scale: "*blue away, red toward*"

baseline—the operator-adjustable dividing line between positive frequency shifts and negative frequency shifts on spectral and color Doppler

Bernoulli's principle—the principle that describes the inverse relationship between velocity and pressure

bidirectional Doppler—the Doppler device that can detect positive and negative Doppler shifts

boundary layer—the stationary layer of blood cells immediately adjacent to the vessel wall

brightness—the term describing the intensity or luminance of the color Doppler display

calf muscle pump—the muscles in the calf that, upon contraction, propel venous blood toward the heart

clutter—acoustic noise in the color and/or spectral Doppler signal

color Doppler imaging (CDI)—Doppler shift information presented as a color (hue) superimposed over the grayscale image

color priority—the setting for color Doppler that allows the operator to select frequency shift threshold; it determines whether color pixels should be displayed preferentially over grayscale pixels

continuity equation—the equation that describes the change in velocity as the area changes in order to maintain the volume of blood flow ($Q = VA$)

continuous-wave (CW) Doppler—Doppler device that uses continuous-wave ultrasound transmission

critical stenosis—the point at which a stenosis is hemodynamically significant with a pressure drop distal to the stenosis

depth ambiguity—the inability to determine the depth of the reflector if the pulses are sent out too fast for them to be timed

diastole—the relaxation of the heart following contraction

directional power Doppler—combination of color Doppler and power Doppler that provides the sensitivity of power Doppler with color Doppler's ability to provide for direction of blood flow

Doppler effect—the change in the frequency of the received signal related to motion of reflector

Doppler equation—the equation that explains the relationship of the Doppler frequency shift (F_D) to the frequency of the transducer (f), the velocity of the blood (v), the angle to blood flow ($\cos \theta$), and the propagation speed (c)

duplex—the real-time 2D imaging combined with the spectral Doppler display

energy gradient—the difference in energy between two points ($E_1 - E_2$)

ensemble length—the number of pulses per scan line in color Doppler; also referred to as "packet size"

Fast Fourier transform (FFT)—a mathematical process used for analyzing and processing the Doppler signal to produce the spectral waveform

flash artifact—a motion artifact caused by the movement of tissue when using power Doppler

flow—the volume of blood per unit time; typically measured in L/min or mL/s; represented by the symbol Q

frequency shift—the difference between the transmitted and received frequencies

friction—a form of resistance; caused by two materials rubbing against each other, thereby converting energy to heat

gravitational potential energy—describes the relationship between gravity, density of the blood, and distance between an arbitrary reference point; also known as "hydrostatic pressure"

hemodynamics—the study of blood flow through the blood vessels of the body

hue—a term used to describe displayed colors (e.g., red, blue, green)

hydrostatic pressure—*see* key term gravitational potential energy

inertia—Newton's principle that states that an object at rest stays at rest and an object in motion stays in motion, unless acted on by an outside force

innervated—supplied with nerves

kinetic energy—the energy form of flowing blood

laminar flow—the flow profile represented by blood that travels in nonmixing layers of different velocities, with the fastest flow in the center and the slowest flow near the vessel walls

law of conservation of energy—the total amount of energy in a system never changes, although it might be in a different form from which it started

luminance—the brightness of the color Doppler image

mm Hg—millimeters of mercury

noise—low-level echoes on the display that do not contribute useful diagnostic information

nondirectional Doppler—Doppler device that cannot differentiate between positive and negative frequency shifts

Nyquist limit—the maximum frequency shift sampled without aliasing; equal to one half the pulse repetition frequency

Ohm's law—a law used in electronics in which flow is equal to the pressure differential divided by resistance

oscillator—the component of a continuous-wave Doppler device that produces the voltage that drives the transducer

packet size—the number of pulses per scan line; also called ensemble length

persistence—the averaging of color frames in order to display blood flow with a low signal-to-noise ratio

phase quadrature—the component of the Doppler device that determines positive opposed to negative frequency shifts and, therefore, direction of blood flow

phasic flow—the characteristic waveform of peripheral veins; flow is determined by respiratory variations as a result of intrathoracic pressure changes

phasicity—in arteries, the phasicity describes shape of the waveform based on the resistiveness of the distal bed (e.g., triphasic, biphasic, monophasic). In veins, phasicity describes the flow pattern that results from respiratory variation

plug flow—the flow profile represented by blood typically flowing at the same velocity

Poiseuille's law—the law that describes the relationship of resistance, pressure, and flow

potential energy—pressure energy created by the beating heart

power Doppler—amplitude mode of Doppler where it is not the shift itself that provides the signal, but the strength (amplitude) of the shift; amplitude is directly proportional to the number of red blood cells

pressure gradient—the difference between pressures at two ends of a blood vessel

pulsatility—blood that flows in a pattern representative of the beating heart, with increases and decreases in pressure and blood flow velocity

pulse repetition frequency—the number of pulses of sound produced in 1 second

pulsed-wave (PW) Doppler—the Doppler technique that uses pulses of sound to obtain Doppler signals from a user-specified depth

range gate—the gate placed by the operator in the region where Doppler sampling is desired; used with pulsed-wave Doppler

range resolution—the ability to determine the depth of echoes by timing how long it takes for the echoes to go from the transducer to the reflector and back; utilized by pulsed-wave devices

Rayleigh scatterers—very small reflectors

resistance—the downstream impedance to flow; determined by vessel length, vessel radius, and viscosity of blood

Reynolds number—the formula used to quantitate the presence of turbulence; Reynolds numbers greater than 2000 typically indicate turbulence

sample volume—the area within the range gate where the Doppler signals are obtained

saturation—the amount of white added to a hue; the more white there is, the less saturated the color

scale—the spectral Doppler and color Doppler tool that controls the number of pulses transmitted per second to obtain the Doppler information; also known as pulse repetition in spectral Doppler and color Doppler

spectral broadening—the filling of the spectral window

spectral window—the area underneath the envelope on the spectral display

stenosis—pathologic narrowing of a blood vessel

sweep speed—the operator-adjustable spectral Doppler control that increases or decreases the number of heartbeats visualized on the spectral display

systole—the time period of the cardiac cycle when the heart is contracting

tardus parvus—an arterial waveform shape with a delayed peak systolic upstroke that indicates proximal obstruction

tissue Doppler imaging (TDI)—color Doppler imaging technique used to image wall motion

transmural pressure—the pressure inside a vessel compared with the pressure outside of a vessel

triplex—the ability to visualize real-time grayscale, color Doppler, and spectral Doppler simultaneously

turbulent flow—chaotic, disorderly flow of blood

variance mode—the color Doppler scale with mean velocities displayed vertically on the scale and turbulence displayed horizontally

vasa vasorum—a network of small blood vessels that supply blood to the walls of arteries and veins

velocity mode—the color Doppler scale with mean velocities displayed vertically

viscous energy—the energy loss caused by friction

wall filter—the operator control that eliminates low-frequency, high-amplitude signals caused by wall or valve motion; also called high-pass filter

z-axis—the brightness, or amplitude, of the dots on the display

HEMODYNAMICS

Types of Energy

Hemodynamics is the study of blood flow through the blood vessels of the body.

It is because of a difference in fluid energy that there is flow through a blood vessel. This difference in fluid energy is called an **energy gradient**, and it is equal to $E_1 - E_2$, where E_1 is the energy at the beginning of the vessel and E_2 is the energy at the end of the vessel. Without an energy gradient, there is no flow.

Pressure energy is the driving force of the blood through the blood vessels. It is the pumping of the heart that provides the necessary **potential energy** at the beginning of the system. Subsequently, this potential energy is converted into **kinetic energy** in the form of flowing blood within the blood vessels (Table 4-1). **Hydrostatic pressure**, also known as **gravitational potential energy**, describes the relationship between gravity, the density of the blood, and the distance between an arbitrary reference point (usually the heart) (Table 4-2).

As blood flows through a vessel, it loses energy. **Viscous energy** is a form of energy loss. It is produced when kinetic energy is converted to heat as a result of **friction**. Blood also undergoes inertial losses, which occur when blood vessels divide, forcing the blood flow to change direction. **Inertia** is described by Newton's first law, which essentially states that an object at rest stays at rest and an object in motion stays in motion, unless acted on by an outside force. Each time blood changes direction, there is an energy loss related to inertia (Table 4-3).

It is important to note that the total energy in a system never changes (the **law of conservation of energy**). That is to say, there must be the same total energy at the end of a vessel as there is at the beginning. However, the types of energy may be different between the two points. For example, potential energy may be the predominant type of energy at the beginning of a vessel, but it is typically converted to kinetic energy and heat (from friction) as the blood travels through the cardiovascular system. The kinetic energy plus the heat energy is equal to the potential energy that was initially found at the beginning of the vessel (Figure 4-1).

Pressure Gradient

Flow is the volume of blood moving through a vessel per unit time. In order for there to be flow, there must be higher pressure at one end of a

TABLE 4-1 Kinetic energy. Kinetic energy is equal to one half of the product of the density (ρ) and the velocity (v) of the blood squared.
Formula
Kinetic energy $= \dfrac{1}{2}\rho v^2$

TABLE 4-2 Hydrostatic pressure. Hydrostatic pressure (P) is equal to the product of the height (h) of the column of blood, the density (ρ) of the blood, and gravity (g).
Formula
$P = \rho g h$

T A B L E 4 - 3 Energy terms related to hemodynamics and their description.	
Terms	**Description**
Potential energy	In the cardiovascular system, the potential energy is created by contraction of the heart. Also referred to as pressure energy.
Kinetic energy	Energy created by flowing blood. The potential energy is converted to kinetic energy minus the energy lost as a result of friction.
Gravitational potential energy	Energy that is created as a result of gravity. In the cardiovascular system, it is the weight of a column of blood. The heaviest pressure is at the bottom of the column because it has to support the weight of blood superior to it. Also known as hydrostatic pressure.
Viscous energy	Energy lost as a result of friction, which occurs when something rubs against something else and heat is created.
Inertial losses	Energy lost as a result of branching of the blood vessels. In order for the blood cells to change direction, some of the initial energy is lost.

blood vessel and lower pressure at the other end. This variance in pressure is referred to as a **pressure gradient** (Table 4-4). The amount of flow in a blood vessel is directly proportional to the pressure gradient. Therefore, the bigger the difference in pressures, the more flow that occurs (Figure 4-2).

Blood Vessels and Blood Flow

Structure of Blood Vessels

Blood vessels are made up of muscle that enables them to expand or contract as needed. The walls of the arteries and veins are similar in that they consist of the same layers. Both arteries and veins have a tunica intima,

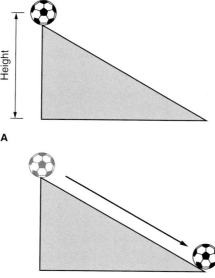

FIGURE 4-1 Potential and kinetic energy. **A.** The ball at the top of the hill has potential energy simply because it has height. **B.** As the ball rolls down the hill, the potential energy is converted into kinetic energy and heat (as a result of friction). The total energy is unchanged.

TABLE 4-4 Pressure gradient. The pressure at the end of the vessel (P_2) is subtracted from the pressure at the beginning of the vessel (P_1).

Formula
$P_1 - P_2$

FIGURE 4-2 Pressure gradient. In image (**A**) the pressure is the same at the beginning of the vessel ($P_1 = 100$ mm Hg) and at the end ($P_2 = 100$ mm Hg). Therefore, there is no pressure gradient and therefore no flow. Image (**B**) depicts a pressure gradient in which there is higher pressure at the beginning ($P_1 = 100$ mm Hg) than at the end of the vessel ($P_2 = 99$ mm Hg). Therefore, there is flow within the vessel.

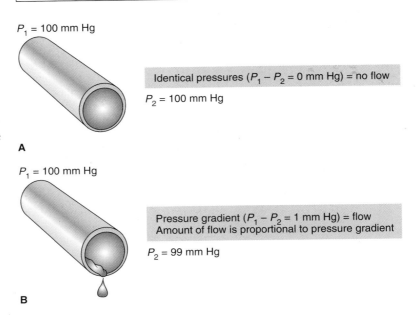

$P_1 = 100$ mm Hg

Identical pressures ($P_1 - P_2 = 0$ mm Hg) = no flow

$P_2 = 100$ mm Hg

A

$P_1 = 100$ mm Hg

Pressure gradient ($P_1 - P_2 = 1$ mm Hg) = flow
Amount of flow is proportional to pressure gradient

$P_2 = 99$ mm Hg

B

tunica media, and tunica adventitia (Table 4-5). The inner layer of the vessel, the layer closest to the flowing blood, is the tunica intima. The outer layer is referred to as the tunica adventitia or externa. This layer requires its own source of blood. The **vasa vasorum**, a small network of blood vessels, accomplishes this task. Between the intima and adventitia is the middle muscular layer, the tunica media. It is this layer of muscle and elastic tissue that differs dramatically between veins and arteries. As blood travels through the cardiovascular system, the arteries and veins experience differences in pressure. Arteries are unique in that they experience a pressure wave as blood is pumped from the heart. One can feel this pressure wave as a "pulse" within the arteries as the heart beats. It is because of this pressure that arteries typically have a much thicker tunica media compared with veins (Figure 4-3).

TABLE 4-5 Layers of the blood vessel walls, their location, and structure.

Layer	Location	Structure
Tunica intima	Inner layer (closest to passing blood)	Made of endothelium
Tunica media	Middle layer	Made of smooth muscle and elastic tissue
Tunica adventitia (externa)	Outermost layer	Made of connective tissue Has its own blood supply via the vasa vasorum

FIGURE 4-3 Blood vessel anatomy. Note the difference in the thickness of the tunica media between an artery (**A**) and a vein (**B**). (Asset provided by Anatomical Chart Co.)

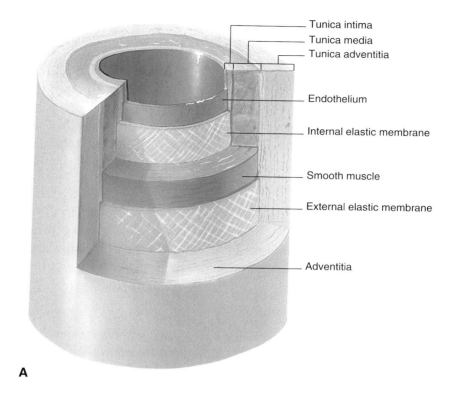

A

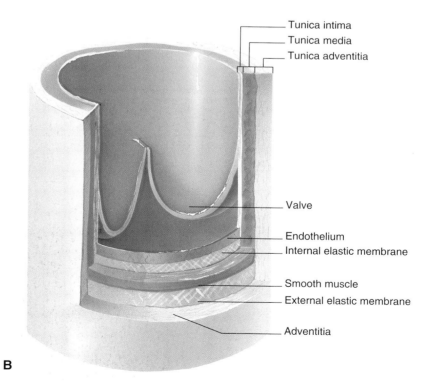

B

Types of Blood Flow

Three types of flow are found in blood vessels: **plug flow**, **laminar flow**, and **turbulent flow**. Plug flow can be found in large blood vessels such as the ascending aorta and at the entrance of vessels such as the common carotid artery (Figure 4-4). The velocity profile of plug flow is blunt as a result of the flow traveling at the same velocity. With plug flow, the blood cells suffer minimal frictional losses at the vessel wall. Plug flow occurs as a result of the acceleration that occurs after **systole**. However, as the blood cells travel through the vessels, friction causes the red blood cells closest to the vessel walls to decrease in velocity, while the fastest velocity is found in the center of the vessel. This velocity profile resembles more of a parabola or is said to have a parabolic shape (Figure 4-5).

Laminar flow, where the red blood cells travel in parallel, nonmixing layers, is the most common type of flow found in arteries. The blood cells that are immediately adjacent to the intima of the vessel are stationary. This region is called the **boundary layer**. Each successive layer extending from the boundary layer inward travels faster than the layer before it, with the fastest flow in the center of the vessel (Figure 4-6).

Turbulent flow results when the red blood cells become chaotic and disorganized, resulting in an assortment of velocities (Figure 4-7). Nonetheless, turbulent flow does not always indicate the presence of pathology. At some points in normal vessels, such as in the area of the carotid bulb, turbulence can be found. Turbulence may also occur from high-velocity flow and from tortuous or kinked vessels. The equation used to quantify the degree of turbulence in a blood vessel is the **Reynolds number** (Table 4-6). A Reynolds number greater than 2000 is considered to represent true turbulence.

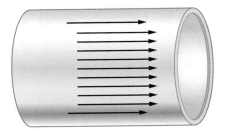

FIGURE 4-4 Plug flow. Plug flow is represented by blood that is typically flowing at the same velocity (*arrows*). Plug flow occurs in large vessels and at the entrance of vessels.

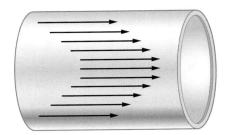

FIGURE 4-5 Laminar flow. Laminar flow is represented by blood that travels in nonmixing layers of different velocities, with the fastest flow in the center and the slowest flow near the vessel walls (*arrows*).

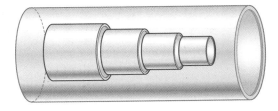

FIGURE 4-6 Layers in laminar flow. The layers of laminar flow are nonmixing concentric layers, with the fastest flow in the center and the slowest flow closest to the vessel walls.

FIGURE 4-7 Turbulent flow and Reynolds number. Flow exiting an area of narrowing will demonstrate turbulence (*curved arrows*). Distal to the obstruction, the flow resumes its prestenotic flow pattern. Reynolds number is used to measure turbulence. Turbulence is present when Reynolds number is greater than 2000.

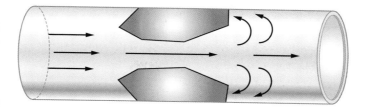

TABLE 4-6 Reynolds number. Reynolds number (*Re*) is defined as the product of the velocity of blood (*v*), two times the radius (*r*) of the vessel, and the density (*ρ*) of the blood divided by the viscosity (*η*) of the blood.
Formula
$Re = \dfrac{v2r\rho}{\eta}$

The Continuity Equation and Bernoulli's Principle

As blood flows through the body, it may encounter vessels that have a decreased radius, possibly secondary to **stenosis** caused by thrombus. When blood flows through an area of decreased radius, the same amount of flow must travel through that area. The **continuity equation** ties together the relationship between the vessel area, the velocity of blood, and the volume of blood flow. The volume of liquid that enters a blood vessel must be the same at any point along the length of the blood vessel (Table 4-7). Blood flow is constant. Therefore, if the area of the vessel decreases, as in the case of a stenosis, the velocity must increase (Figure 4-8). Putting a finger over the

TABLE 4-7 Continuity equation. The volume of liquid that enters a blood vessel must be the same at any point along the length of the blood vessel. The continuity equation demonstrates the relationship between velocity (*V*) and area (*A*). Flow (*Q*) is equal to the product of velocity and area.
Formula
$Q = VA$

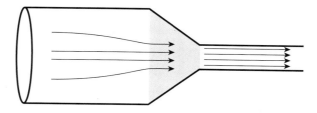

A

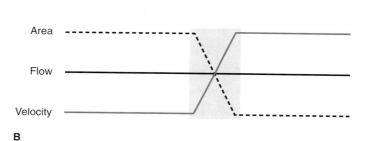

FIGURE 4-8 Continuity equation explains the relationship between area, flow, and velocity. Blood flow (*arrow*) through a blood vessel (**A**). There is an increase in velocity as the area decreases in the region of the narrowing of the vessel (**B**). The volume of flow does not change.

B

FIGURE 4-9 Bernoulli's principle. Bernoulli's principle can be demonstrated by taking two sheets of paper and placing one on top of the other. While holding the paper together toward your mouth, blow between them. Notice that the sheets are drawn toward each other. The reason that the sheets are drawn together demonstrates Bernoulli's principle. That is, as the velocity of air between the sheets of paper increases, there is a pressure drop between them and they are drawn toward each other.

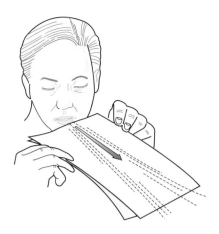

front of a garden hose demonstrates the continuity equation. The area at the outlet of the hose decreases, so the velocity must increase in order to maintain flow. **Bernoulli's principle** states that an increase in velocity must be accompanied by a corresponding decrease in pressure. This inverse relationship between pressure and velocity is linked to the law of conservation of energy. Subsequently, any increase in velocity is an increase in energy, and therefore something (the pressure) must decrease to preserve the total energy. Once the vessel goes back to its prestenotic area, there is a decrease in velocity with a corresponding increase in pressure. Using the previous example of a water hose, although the water that was shooting out of the hose was at a higher velocity than it was at preobstruction, it was at a lower pressure than that of the water entering the hose. Bernoulli's principle is further explained in Figure 4-9. The formula for Bernoulli's principle is provided in Table 4-8.

Poiseuille's Law

In addition to the pressure differential, there are other factors that may increase or decrease the amount of blood flowing through a blood vessel, including the length of the vessel, the radius of the vessel, and the viscosity of the blood. These factors are all tied together by an equation known as **Poiseuille's law** (Tables 4-9 and 4-10). Poiseuille's law describes the relationship between the volume of blood flow and the **resistance** to flow in a blood vessel. Essentially, the law states that flow is equal to the difference in pressure divided by the resistance to flow in the vessel. As stated by the formulas in Tables 4-9 and 4-10, if the length of the vessel or the viscosity of the blood (both of which contribute to resistance to flow) increases, there is decreased flow. Likewise, if the radius of the vessel increases, flow increases. In fact, if the radius doubles, flow increases by a factor of 16. In summary, an increase in length or viscosity decreases flow, while an increase in radius increases flow.

T A B L E **4 - 8** Bernoulli's principle. ΔP represents the pressure gradient ($P_1 - P_2$) and v is the velocity of the blood through a stenosis.
Formula
$\Delta P = 4v^2$

TABLE 4-9 Poiseuille's law (short form). Flow (Q) is equal to the difference in pressure (ΔP) divided by the resistance (R) to flow in the vessel. R is the resistance and L is the length of the vessel. The η in the equation represents the viscosity of the blood and r is the radius of the vessel.

Formula
$Q = \dfrac{\Delta P}{R}$ where $R = \dfrac{8L\eta}{\pi r^4}$

TABLE 4-10 Poiseuille's law (long form). Combination of the two previous equations into one equation. (See Table 4-9 for explanation of abbreviations.)

Formula
$Q = \dfrac{\Delta P \pi r^4}{8L\eta}$

Inertial losses occur as vessels branch and change direction. Friction, another form of resistance, is the loss of energy in the form of heat and is another detriment to flow. As the arterioles branch out into capillaries, frictional and inertial losses are responsible for the accompanying decrease in the velocity of the blood. The capillaries are tiny, typically about the width of a red blood cell. It is the small size of the capillaries that contributes to the energy loss and slow velocity of flow. However, this slow flow is essential for the function of the capillaries, which is the exchange of nutrients and waste products.

Poiseuille's law assumes a straight (noncurved), rigid (nonelastic) pipe with a steady flow rate (nonpulsatile). Unfortunately, this does not describe the blood vessels found in the human body. Although there is no simple way to describe the cardiovascular system, Poiseuille's law demonstrates the relationships of flow and resistance. Poiseuille's law is analogous to **Ohm's law**, a principle in electronics in which flow is equal to the pressure differential divided by resistance (Table 4-11).

Resistance and Stenotic Flow

The theorems provided by Bernoulli and Poiseuille describe the energy losses and changes in energy that occur as blood travels. It has been previously described that flow is a constant and does not change. Said another way, the heart continues to beat and pump the same volume of blood regardless of the presence of a stenosis downstream. However, there can be a stenosis so severe that it compromises flow to a certain part of the body. A **critical stenosis**, also referred to as a hemodynamically significant stenosis,

---

TABLE 4-11 Ohm's law. Ohm's law is a principle in electronics in which flow (I, or current) is equal to the pressure differential (V, or voltage) divided by resistance (R).

Formula
$I = \dfrac{V}{R}$

FIGURE 4-10 Vessel arrangement and effective resistance. Blood vessels may be connected end to end (**A**) or flow into multiple parallel channels (**B**). The effective resistance, the resistance of the distal bed, is the sum of the individual resistances when multiple vessels are connected in series (**A**). The equation that represents vessels in series is: $R = R_1 + R_2 + R_3 \uparrow$. When vessels are connected in parallel (**B**), the effective resistance is reduced, as there are more channels or paths for the flow to go, or $R = 1/R_1 + 1/R_2 + 1/R_3 \uparrow$.

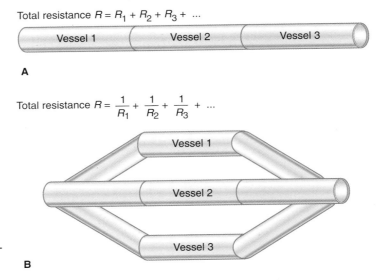

Total resistance $R = R_1 + R_2 + R_3 + \dots$

Vessel 1 | Vessel 2 | Vessel 3

A

Total resistance $R = \dfrac{1}{R_1} + \dfrac{1}{R_2} + \dfrac{1}{R_3} + \dots$

Vessel 1

Vessel 2

Vessel 3

B

is one in which there is decreased distal flow. This situation would lead to a significant pressure gradient. A cross-sectional area loss of 75% is generally considered to be hemodynamically significant, though this percentage may vary among vessels. It is important to remember that a 75% decrease in area corresponds to a 50% decrease in diameter.

Blood vessels may be connected end to end (in series) or flow into multiple parallel channels (in parallel) (Figure 4-10). The effective resistance, the resistance of the distal bed, is the sum of the individual resistances when multiple vessels are connected in series (Table 4-12). When vessels are connected in parallel, the effective resistance is reduced, as there are more channels or paths for flow to exploit (Table 4-13 and Figure 4-11). Arterioles, because of their muscular walls, are the main contributors to the resistance in the cardiovascular system. The **innervated** arteriole walls can constrict or dilate in response to signals from the brain to either increase or decrease flow distally.

At the region of a subcritical stenosis, the velocity of the blood cells must increase in order to maintain the same volume flow. The area of increased velocity is accompanied by a decrease in pressure through this

TABLE 4-12 Vessels in series. The effective resistance (R), the resistance of the distal bed, is the sum of the individual resistances when multiple vessels are connected in series.
Formula
$R = R_1 + R_2 + R_3 + \uparrow$

TABLE 4-13 Vessels in parallel. The effective resistance (R) is reduced, as there are more channels or paths for blood to access.
Formula
$R = 1/R_1 + 1/R_2 + 1/R_3 + \uparrow$

FIGURE 4-11 Example of effective resistance. A simple comparison for in-series and in-parallel vessels is that of trying to leave an island that has only one bridge. When many cars are trying to leave the island at the same time on one bridge "in-series," the resistance to the flow of traffic is high (**A**). When more bridges are opened (**B**), the cars are able to travel out of the city quite rapidly "in-parallel," because there is little or low resistance to the flow of traffic.

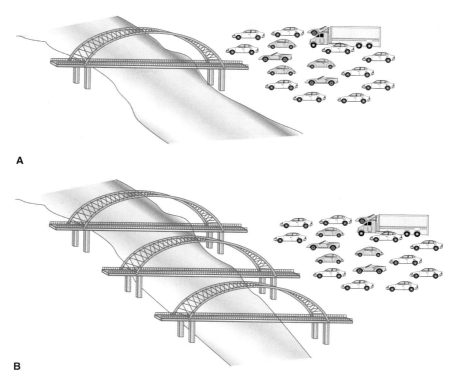

region, as described by the Bernoulli's principle. As the blood exits the region of narrowing and enters a suddenly expanded vessel, there is turbulence as the blood spills out. This turbulence eventually dissipates and downstream the flow returns to its previous prestenotic state. Another important hemodynamic concept is as follows: with a stenosis, it is more detrimental to have two stenoses in series than a single lesion because there is more of an energy loss with two stenoses in series.

It is vital to recognize that blood will always follow the path of least resistance. If a major highway is blocked because of an obstruction, like an accident, the cars will exit the highway and drive through side streets, eventually rejoining the highway past the accident location. In the body, if a major artery is blocked it becomes the path of highest resistance, while the previously collapsed collaterals become the path of least resistance. The higher pressure proximal to a stenosis causes the collaterals to open up and the blood follows the lower-resistance path. Distal to the stenosis, the collateral eventually rejoins the main artery. In chronic disease, if the collateral network is extensive enough, the net flow distal to the stenosis may actually be normal (Figure 4-12). Collaterals are formed over time and in response to chronic change. They are typically not found in the presence of an acute obstruction.

Venous Hemodynamics and Hydrostatic Pressure

As flow leaves the capillaries, it enters the larger venules. The veins that are located between the capillaries and the right atrium of the heart get progressively wider, thus offering lower resistance to flow. The pressure in the venules is very low, about 15 millimeters of mercury (**mm Hg**), but still higher than the pressure in the right atrium, which is typically 0 to 8 mm Hg.

FIGURE 4-12 Collateral flow. **A.** In the presence of normal unobstructed flow, collateral is a relatively high-pressure vessel because of its small radius, whereas the larger vessel provides the normal low-pressure pathway. **B.** In the presence of an obstruction (*arrow*), the larger vessel becomes the high-resistance pathway. The increased pressure causes the collateral to dilate, thereby increasing its radius and decreasing its pressure. The collateral essentially becomes the path of least resistance.

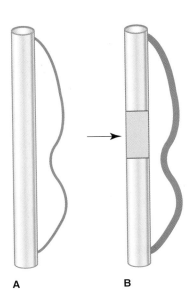

A   B

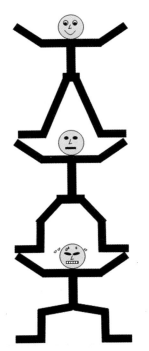

FIGURE 4-13 Hydrostatic pressure. This image demonstrates the effect of hydrostatic pressure. When three people are standing on each other's shoulders, the person at the bottom has to support the most weight while the person at the top has it relatively easy.

Assuming that the person is supine, this small, but still significant difference in pressure is a pressure gradient, and therefore, there exists forward flow (toward the heart).

When someone is in the standing position, gravity acts on the blood in the form of hydrostatic pressure. As mentioned earlier in this chapter, hydrostatic pressure is the weight of a column of fluid from a certain reference point. In the humans, that reference point is the heart, the point at which the hydrostatic pressure is zero. Below the heart, the weight of this column of blood increases with the distance from the heart (Figure 4-13). Blood in a vertical tube acts in the same way. That is, the farther from the heart, the more weight there is to support. Therefore, the highest hydrostatic pressures are located at more distal parts of the body, such as the feet and ankles. Hydrostatic pressure is the reason that venous stasis ulcers are found at the ankles and not in the thighs.

Recall that hydrostatic pressure can be calculated by using the density of the blood, gravity, and the height at which you are measuring, or distance from the heart (Table 4-2). Notice in the formula that the height variable is the only variable that is not a constant. If the point at which you are measuring is below the heart, the hydrostatic pressure will be positive. Conversely, if a point is measured above the heart, such as an outstretched arm over the head, the hydrostatic pressure will be negative (Figures 4-14 and 4-15).

Appropriate venous return to the heart requires several mechanisms to work properly (Table 4-14). First, as mentioned early, a pressure gradient exists between the venules and the right atrium. Second, with inspiration an area of low pressure is formed within the thorax, causing the blood to be forced into the chest. Third, venous valves, folds of endothelial tissue inside of the veins, provide a method to ensure forward flow by only permitting the flow of blood in one direction, to the heart. The **calf muscle pump** provides the final mechanism. The soleal sinuses inside the calf muscle store venous blood. When the calf muscles are used, blood is forced into the veins.

FIGURE 4-14 Change in hydrostatic pressure in the extremities as a result of position. When the arm is held below the heart, hydrostatic pressure increases and veins dilate within the hand and fill with blood (**A**). When the hand is raised over the head, the hydrostatic pressure is negative and the veins collapse (**B**).

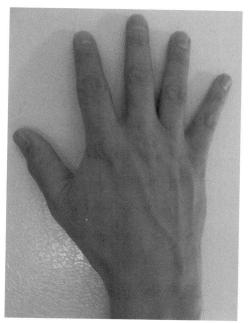
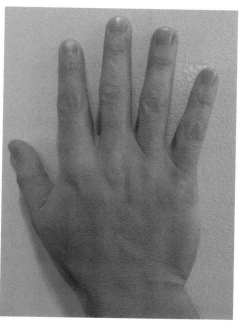

A   **B**

FIGURE 4-15 Hydrostatic pressure and the heart. If the point at which you are measuring is below the heart, the hydrostatic pressure will be positive. Conversely, if a point is measured above the heart, such as an outstretched arm over the head, the hydrostatic pressure will be negative.

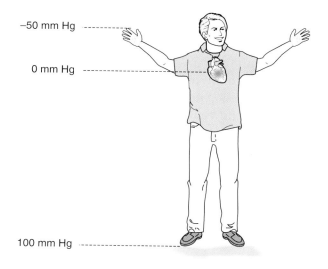

−50 mm Hg

0 mm Hg

100 mm Hg

TABLE 4-14	Mechanism of venous return to the heart.
Mechanism	**Explanation**
Pressure gradient	There is a small but significant pressure gradient between the venules and the right atrium of the heart.
Venous valves	Functional venous valves keep the blood flowing in the proper direction: toward the heart.
Calf muscle pump	Contraction of the calf muscles propels blood from the soleal sinuses in the calf toward the heart.
Intrathoracic pressure changes	Inspiration causes a negative pressure in the thorax, essentially sucking the blood toward the heart.

FIGURE 4-16 Transmural pressure. In the supine position, the vein takes on an elliptical shape due to low transmural pressure (**A**). In the standing position, the vein takes on a circular shape due to high transmural pressure (**B**).

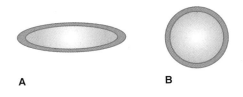

FIGURE 4-17 Phasicity of the peripheral venous form. **A.** Phasic flow indicates respiratory variability. **B.** Continuous flow implies intrinsic or extrinsic obstruction between sampled vessel and the heart.

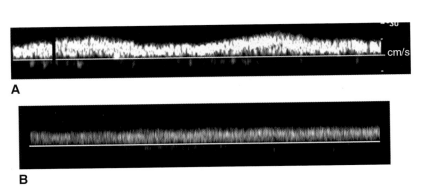

There is not only pressure inside the veins, but outside the veins as well in the form of extrinsic pressure. **Transmural pressure** is the difference between the pressure inside the vein (intravascular pressure) and the surrounding tissue. With low transmural pressure, which may occur when a patient is lying supine, the force outside the vein exceeds the pressure inside the vein and the vein collapses and has an elliptical shape. When the patient stands and the hydrostatic pressure increases, the transmural pressure increases and the vein assumes a circular shape (Figure 4-16).

Flow in the veins should not be pulsatile, with the exception of the systemic veins in close proximity to the heart. Rather, veins should be **phasic** or show variations that relate to respiration. **Pulsatility** in the peripheral veins may indicate trouble with the right side of the patient's heart and should be documented. Lack of respiratory phasicity, referred to as "continuous flow," may be an indicator of intrinsic thrombus or extrinsic compression between the vein being sampled and the heart and should also be documented (Figure 4-17).

Pulsatility and Phasicity

Unlike veins, arteries should be pulsatile in nature, with a distinct **systole** and **diastole** that correspond to both the flow from the heart and to the distal vascular bed. Flow is often described by the shape of its waveform on spectral Doppler as triphasic, biphasic (collectively known as "multiphasic"), or monophasic (Figure 4-18). Flow that is triphasic or biphasic feeds a high-resistance bed, and there is typically little diastolic flow evident, with possibly some flow reversal in diastole. Monophasic flow feeds a low-resistance bed. A low-resistance bed is a bed that demands constant flow in all phases of the cardiac cycle. Examples of a low-resistance bed are the internal carotid artery (ICA), which feeds the brain, and the renal artery that supplies the kidney. The shape of the waveform may be an indicator of disease that is more distal or more proximal to the sampling point. In the presence of a proximal stenosis, the distal arterioles will dilate, thereby allowing more oxygenated blood to get to the periphery. The increase in diameter of the vessels is accompanied by a pressure drop. For example, the lower extremity arteries are

FIGURE 4-18 Types of arterial flow. **A.** Triphasic flow. **B.** Biphasic flow. **C.** Monophasic flow.

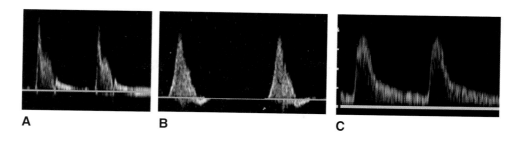

A   B   C

normally high-resistance vessels. However, if there is a proximal femoral artery (FA) obstruction, there will be dilatation of the distal arterioles, with a corresponding change to monophasic flow in the spectral waveform of the FA.

Arterial **phasicity** is always about the resistance in the distal bed. For example, in the resting patient, monophasic flow is always abnormal in the lower extremities. If monophasic flow is seen in the lower extremity arteries of the resting patient, it indicates persistent dilatation downstream, an abnormal condition. Conversely, blood vessels that normally have low-resistance waveforms, such as the ICA, should never exhibit a high-resistance pattern. If high-resistance flow is noted in the ICA, it would be an ominous sign indicating a distal high-pressure state, as seen with distal occlusion or near occlusion, cerebral edema, or brain death.

An additional noteworthy waveform shape that can be indicative of pathology is **tardus parvus**, which is seen in the presence of a proximal obstruction (Figure 4-19). Tardus parvus waveforms are identified by a delay in the upstroke of the systolic component of the waveform (time-to-peak). Most arteries have flow that initially accelerates rapidly, causing a sharp systolic upstroke. An increased acceleration time, represented by a delay in the systolic upstroke, is a sign that there is an obstruction, and that obstruction is located more proximal to the point of sampling. It is important to remember that a proximal obstruction causes distal arteriolar dilatation; therefore, tardus parvus waveforms are monophasic in nature.

Effects of Exercise on Flow

In the resting patient, the peripheral lower extremity arteries are normally of high resistance due to distal arteriolar constriction. With exercise, there is an increased demand for oxygen by the muscles. This increase in demand causes arteriolar dilatation, which results in larger-diameter blood vessels, and therefore a lower-resistance distal bed with a corresponding increase in blood flow. In the normal patient, there is little pressure change in the distal lower extremities as a result of this arteriolar dilatation. The patient with arterial obstructive disease may have normal resting pressures, but the increased demand for oxygen that occurs with exercise may be more than the blood vessels are able to supply, causing a pressure drop distally.

FIGURE 4-19 Tardus parvus waveform. This image of a tardus parvus waveform demonstrates a delayed upstroke (increased acceleration time).

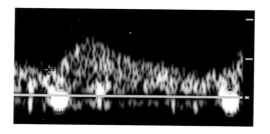

DOPPLER PRINCIPLES

The Doppler Effect

The effect of differing frequencies with motion was first noted by Christian Doppler and is thus called the **Doppler effect**. Doppler discovered that when sound impinges on a stationary reflector, the reflected frequency is identical to the transmitted, or incident, frequency. However, when a reflector is moving toward the transducer, the reflected frequency will be higher than the transmitted frequency. Likewise, when a reflector is moving away from the transducer, the reflected frequency will be lower than the transmitted frequency (Figure 4-20). The difference between the transmitted and reflected frequencies is called the **frequency shift**, or Doppler shift. A positive frequency shift occurs when a reflector is moving in a direction that is toward the transducer. A negative frequency shift occurs when a reflector is moving in a direction that is away from the transducer. The frequency shift can be calculated by utilizing the **Doppler equation** (Table 4-15 and Figure 4-21).

When the transmitted frequency is subtracted from the reflected frequency, the result is a number that is approximately 1/1000th of the operating

FIGURE 4-20 Frequency shifts and moving reflector. **A.** With a stationary reflector, the reflected frequency is equal to the incident frequency, resulting in no change in frequency. **B.** With a reflector moving toward the source, the reflected frequency is greater than the incident frequency, resulting in a positive frequency shift. **C.** With a reflector moving away from the source, the reflected frequency is less than the incident frequency, resulting in a negative frequency shift.

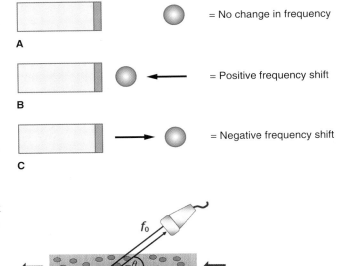

A   = No change in frequency

B   = Positive frequency shift

C   = Negative frequency shift

FIGURE 4-21 Doppler shift diagram. Calculation of the Doppler shift requires knowledge of the transmitted frequency (f_0), the reflected frequency (f_r), the angle of incidence (θ), and the speed of sound. See text for details. (Image reprinted with permission from Feigenbaum H. Feigenbaum's Echocardiography, 6th Ed. Philadelphia, PA: Lippincott Williams & Wilkins, 2004.)

T A B L E 4 - 1 5 **The Doppler equation. In the formula, the frequency shift (F_D) in measured in Hertz by the ultrasound machine. The frequency shift is the difference between the incident frequency and the reflected frequency. The product of the operating frequency (f) of the transducer multiplied by 2, the velocity (v) of the blood, and the cosine (cos θ) of the Doppler angle is divided by the propagation speed (c) of sound through soft tissue.**

Formula
$F_D = \dfrac{2\,f v \cos\theta}{c}$

FIGURE 4-22 How to calculate frequency shift. The Doppler frequency shift is equal to the reflected frequency minus the transmitted frequency. If the result, which is in the audible range of sound, is a positive number, then the flow is moving toward the transducer. If the result is a negative number, then the flow is moving away from the transducer.

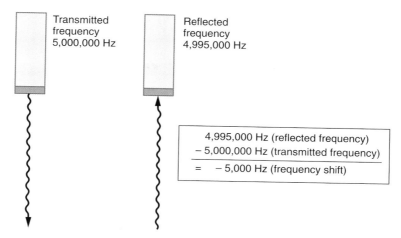

Transmitted frequency 5,000,000 Hz

Reflected frequency 4,995,000 Hz

4,995,000 Hz (reflected frequency)
− 5,000,000 Hz (transmitted frequency)
= − 5,000 Hz (frequency shift)

frequency. The resultant value is in the audible range of sound, meaning that all that is needed to hear the frequency shift is a set of speakers or headphones. If the resultant value is a positive number, then there is a positive shift and flow is moving toward the transducer. Likewise, if the resultant value is a negative number, then there is a negative shift and flow is moving away from the transducer (Figure 4-22).

While the frequency shift is measured by the machine, it is the velocity of the blood that is of interest to the imager, and not the frequency shift itself. The ultrasound system measures the frequency shift but calculates the velocity (Table 4-16).

Doppler works because the incident sound reflects off of the red blood cells in the blood. Red blood cells are small, normally about 7.0 μm. Because of their size, they are natural **Rayleigh scatterers**. Rayleigh scatterers are very small compared with the incident wavelength. As frequency increases, the intensity of scatter increases proportional to the fourth power of the frequency; therefore, a small increase in frequency results in a dramatic increase in scatter (Figure 4-23). Higher-frequency transducers may

FIGURE 4-23 Scatter. The higher the frequency, the more scatter there is. Scatter, a form of attenuation, keeps the beam from penetrating. The more energy that is scattered the less there is to penetrate deeper in the body.

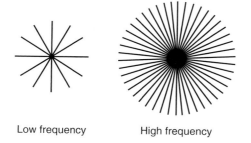

Low frequency   High frequency

TABLE **4 - 1 6** Formula for velocity. Velocity (*v*) is equal to the product of the propagation speed of sound through soft tissue (*c*) and the frequency shift (F_D), divided by the product of the operating frequency (*f*) multiplied by 2 and the cosine (cos θ) of the Doppler angle.
Formula
$$v = \frac{cF_D}{2f \cos \theta}$$

TABLE 4-17	Cosines of the angles.
Angle	**Cosine of the Angle**
0°	1.0
30°	0.87
45°	0.71
60°	0.50
90°	0.00

provide stronger Doppler signals, but at the expense of the attenuation. Therefore, the higher the frequency, the more scatter there is, and therefore, the more attenuation. Remember that scatter is a form of attenuation. Therefore, if the energy is scattered, it is not transmitted deeper into the tissue. Essentially, there has to be a trade-off between improved resolution and penetration.

In the Doppler equation, it is not the Doppler angle that is utilized in the equation, but rather the cosine of the angle (Table 4-17). As the Doppler angle increases, the cosine of the angle decreases. That is, the Doppler angle and the frequency shift are inversely proportional. The Doppler angle must be known in order to accurately calculate the velocities, although in echocardiography a 0° angle is always assumed. Table 4-17 reveals that the cosine of 0 is 1. If "1" is plugged into the Doppler equation, the equation would not change at all. Therefore, the most accurate Doppler shift (and therefore the most accurate velocity) will come from a 0° angle. Because of the inverse relationship between the Doppler angle and the cosine of the angle, as the angle increases the frequency shift decreases. Therefore, the highest Doppler shift comes from a 0° angle. No Doppler shift is obtained at a 90° angle; at an angle of 90°, the cosine of 90 is 0, and therefore, the Doppler shift is 0.

Some Doppler devices are **nondirectional**, or unable to distinguish between positive or negative Doppler shifts. In order to determine the direction of flow, Doppler devices use **phase quadrature** to determine whether there is a positive shift, flow toward the transducer, or a negative shift, flow away from the transducer. Phase quadrature permits **bidirectional Doppler**, which is able to display positive versus negative shifts. There are two ways of obtaining a Doppler signal: continuous-wave (CW) and pulsed-wave (PW).

Continuous-Wave Doppler

A **continuous-wave (CW) Doppler** device consists of two elements. One element is used by the system to constantly transmit sound and the other is used to constantly receive sound. CW devices are constructed this way because the piezoelectric elements used by the system to create ultrasound cannot send and receive at the same time. CW devices do not pause to listen for the return echo. Nor do they calculate how long it takes for the echo to return. Therefore, CW devices have no **range resolution**, or the ability to determine how far away the reflectors are from the transducer. It is for this reason that CW transducers themselves do not provide a 2D image, only a spectral Doppler waveform (see the section "Analyzing the Spectral Waveform"). The **sample volume**, or region that is being measured by Doppler, is very large with CW Doppler. Any blood vessel that lies within the sample volume will be measured and displayed in the signal. With CW Doppler, the operator is not able to select a specific vessel. This dilemma can present problems when there are several vessels within the sample volume.

The CW transducer is driven by an oscillator that provides a continuous voltage to the transmitting element. With CW transducers, the oscillating voltage is equal to the operating frequency. If the **oscillator** vibrates at 3,000,000 times per second, the CW transducer operates at 3 MHz. The signal processor in the machine compares the transmitted and received frequencies, and their difference is sent to a loudspeaker and/or spectrum analyzer. It is also important to remember that there is no damping with a CW transducer; if the sound is being transmitted continuously, damping is not needed. The continuously transmitting CW device has a 100% transmit time. Therefore, the duty factor of a CW device is 100%, or 1.

Analyzing the Spectral Waveform

The signal that is received by the transducer is a complex mix of frequency shifts and time. The signal undergoes processing before it is displayed to improve the analysis of Doppler information. Spectral analysis dismantles the complex signal and breaks it down by frequency. The resultant waveform is a visual, quantifiable representation of what is happening in the blood vessel at a given point in time. The mathematical technique used to break down the signal and produce a spectral waveform is called **Fast Fourier Transform (FFT)**. Accurate velocity measurements are needed to be able to quantify the level of disease and perform other assessments, and it is FFT that accomplishes this task. The spectral display provides the following information: time, velocity, frequency shift, flow direction, and amplitude (Figure 4-24).

Time is displayed on the spectral display along the x-axis. Tick marks represent seconds, so it is possible to calculate events as they occur over a specific period of time. The number of seconds displayed at one time can be adjusted by changing the **sweep speed** of the Doppler instrument (Figure 4-25).

As stated earlier, it is the frequency shift that is measured by the machine; however, it is the velocity information that is of most interest. Therefore,

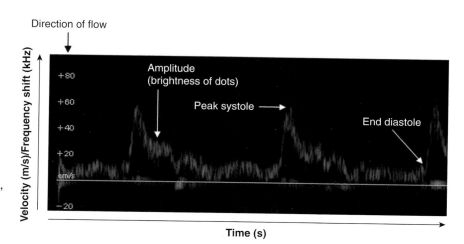

FIGURE 4-24 Spectral waveform. The spectral display provides the following information: time, velocity, frequency shift, flow direction, and amplitude.

FIGURE 4-25 Changing the sweep speed. The sweep speed can be changed to display more (**A**) or fewer (**B**) waveforms on the screen at one time.

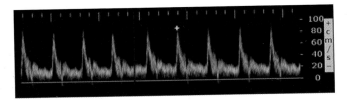

A

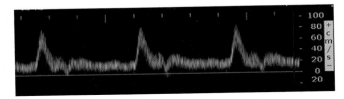

B

today's spectral displays commonly display only velocity information. On some machines, it may be possible to also display frequency shift information, but to reduce interoperator variability, angle-corrected velocities are commonly used (except in echocardiography, which assumes 0° angles).

Measurement of the flow velocity enables the sonographer to measure peak systolic and end diastolic measurements, which are, in turn, used to quantify the degree of disease within vessels. In addition to the peak systolic and end diastolic velocities, the mean velocity is used for some applications. The mean velocity is derived by tracing the spectral waveform from end diastole of one heartbeat to end diastole of the next heartbeat. Examples of measurements that are obtained on a spectral waveform include the resistive index (RI) and the pulsatility index (PI). The RI is used to quantitate the resistiveness of the distal bed (Table 4-18 and Figure 4-26). An

TABLE 4-18 Formula for resistive index. In this formula for resistive index (RI), peak systolic velocity (A) is subtracted from the end diastolic velocity (B) and then divided by the peak systolic velocity.
Formula
$$RI = \frac{A - B}{A}$$

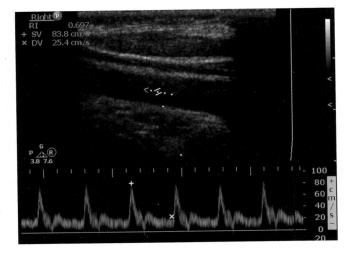

FIGURE 4-26 Resistive index. This image demonstrates the measurement obtained for the resistive index.

TABLE 4-19 The formula for pulsatility index. In this formula of pulsatility index (PI), the peak systolic velocity (A) is subtracted from the end diastolic velocity (B) and then divided by the *mean* or average of the velocities between peak systole and end diastole.
Formula
$$PI = \frac{A-B}{Mean}$$

example of the use of RI is for the analysis of the kidneys in cases of hydronephrosis. The PI is used to determine how pulsatile a vessel is over time (Table 4-19 and Figure 4-27). The PI is often used in obstetrics in evaluation of fetal brain and umbilical cord. Both of these measurements endeavor to estimate the relative difference between systole and diastole.

Flow direction is displayed on the spectral display as flow being above or below the baseline. Flow on one side of the baseline is a "positive shift" and flow on the other side represents a "negative shift." The flow can be inverted for convention so that flow always appears above the baseline, even when it represents a negative shift. The spectral display also allows for display of pathologic reversal of flow. Reversal of flow may occur in the ICAs when cerebral edema is present, or in the fetal umbilical artery when there is severe placental insufficiency.

When trying to determine whether the flow is "toward" or "away" from the transducer, the practitioner must search for the minus (negative) sign that precedes the velocity on the spectral velocity chart. Some machines display "INVERTED" instead of a minus sign to denote that the display has been inverted (Figure 4-28).

The amplitude of the signal is represented by the brightness of the dots on the spectral display, the so-called **z-axis**. The brighter the dots of the spectral waveform, the more red blood cells that make up the signal (Figure 4-29).

The envelope of the waveform represents how many red blood cells are traveling at that velocity at a specific period in time (Figure 4-30). The wider the range of velocities in a sample in a given point of time, the thicker the envelope. In a normal vessel, a small sample volume is typically used in order to sample only the highest velocities in the center of the vessel. A large sample volume that encompasses both the fast central flow and all the

FIGURE 4-27 Pulsatility index. This image demonstrates the measurement obtained for the pulsatility index.

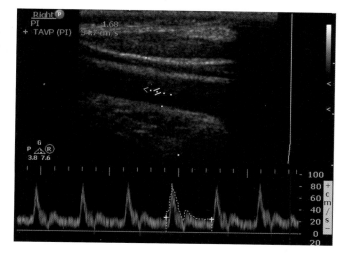

FIGURE 4-28
Demonstration of a negative frequency shift. Some manufacturers signify negative frequency shifts by placing a minus sign (*arrow*) in front of the velocities on the Doppler scale (**A**), whereas others signify a negative frequency shift by displaying the word "inverted" (*arrow*) above the spectral waveform (**B**).

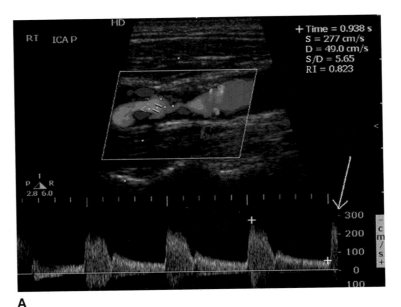

A

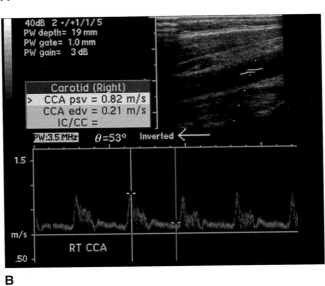

B

FIGURE 4-29 Amplitude of the Doppler signal. The less bright the spectral waveform, the fewer the red blood cells that make up the image (**A**). The brighter the dots of the spectral waveform, the more red blood cells that make up the signal (**B**).

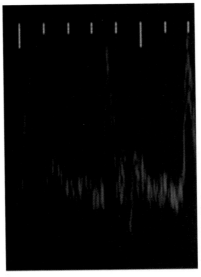

A

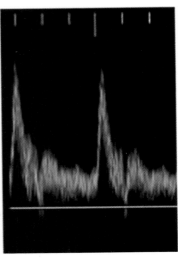

B

FIGURE 4-30 The envelope and window of the spectral display. The envelope (*envelope*) of the waveform represents how many red blood cells are traveling at that velocity at a specific period in time. The spectral window (*window*) is the area under the envelope.

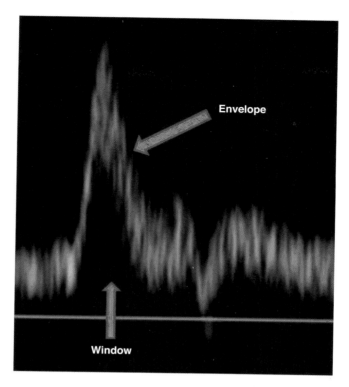

progressively decreasing velocities toward the edges will represent many different velocities (Figure 4-31). The area under the envelope is called the **spectral window**. A flow sample in which the red blood cells are traveling at almost identical speeds, as in the case of laminar flow with a small sample volume, will demonstrate a thin envelope. Conversely, only analyzing one instance of time in turbulent flow or utilizing when a large sample volume it used will demonstrate a wide range of velocities. This turbulent flow therefore demonstrates a filling-in of the spectral envelope. This is termed **spectral broadening** (Figure 4-31). As mentioned earlier, turbulence is not always pathologic. Turbulence is normal and expected in some instances, such as in the area of the carotid bulb. However, if turbulence is seen where one expects to see laminar flow, further investigation is warranted. The spectral window disappears in the presence of spectral broadening. CW flow uses a large sample volume and samples many vessels (at a variety of velocities) at the same time. Therefore, CW waveforms will typically demonstrate spectral broadening (Figure 4-32).

Pulsed-Wave Doppler

Pulsed-wave (PW) Doppler functions much like PW grayscale imaging in that it transmits pulses of sound and waits for the sound to return in order to determine the depth of the returning echoes (Figure 4-33).

Unlike CW, PW Doppler allows the operator to select the depth at which the Doppler measurements will be taken. The operator places a **range gate** over the vessel to be sampled, and the area within that gate, the sample volume, is where the PW Doppler signal is obtained. The operator can select the size of the sample volume by adjusting a "gate" control on the machine,

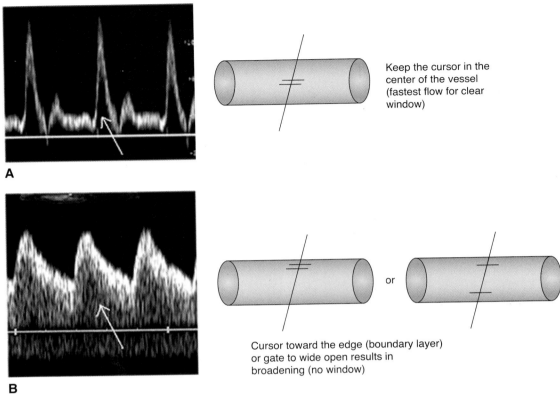

FIGURE 4-31 Sample volume size and appearance of the spectral waveform. **A.** A small sample volume placed in the center of a vessel where flow is the fastest will result in a clear window (*arrow*). **B.** A large sample or one taken near a vessel wall will demonstrate spectral broadening of the window (*arrow*).

FIGURE 4-32 Spectral broadening with CW Doppler. Note the filling in of the spectral window (*arrow*).

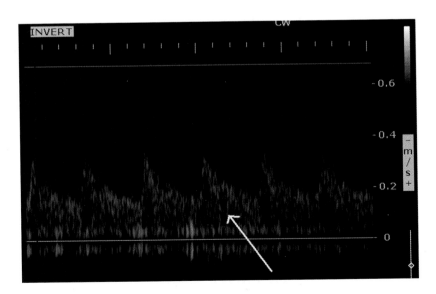

which permits many different size sample volumes (Figure 4-34). Grayscale devices typically use 2 to 3 cycles per pulse to produce a B-mode image. PW Doppler devices typically transmit anywhere from 5 to 30 cycles per pulse. This higher pulse length provides a more accurate sampling of the blood.

PW Doppler also utilizes **angle correct**. Angle correction is used with PW Doppler in order to more accurately calculate the velocities from the

FIGURE 4-33 Pulsed-wave and continuous-wave Doppler. Pulsed-wave, also referred to as PW Doppler, much like pulsed-wave grayscale imaging, transmits pulses of sound and waits for the sound to return in order to determine the depth of the returning echoes. A continuous-wave, or CW Doppler device, consists of two elements. One element is used by the system to constantly transmit sound and the other is used to constantly receive sound. (Image reprinted with permission from Feigenbaum H. Feigenbaum's Echocardiography, 6th Ed. Philadelphia, PA: Lippincott Williams & Wilkins, 2004.)

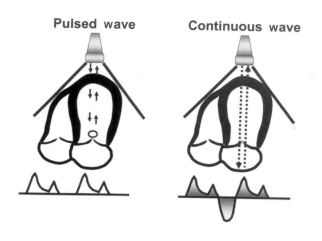

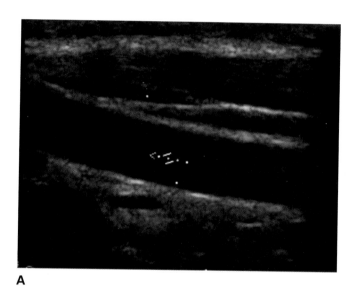

A

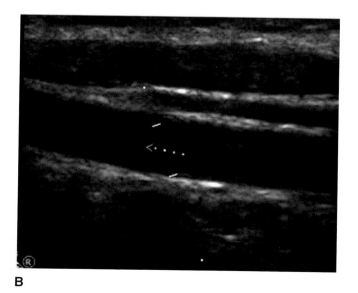

FIGURE 4-34 Controlling the size of the sample volume. A small pulsed-wave sample volume can be placed in the center of the vessel (**A**). The sample volume can also be larger if needed (**B**).

B

FIGURE 4-35 Duplex Doppler. Pulsed-wave Doppler devices also permit duplex imaging, where the B-mode image is on the display at the same time as the Doppler signal.

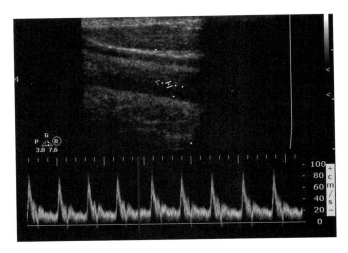

frequency shifts. When performing Doppler studies, it is rare that the transducer is parallel to the flowing blood. Therefore, angle correction is used to inform the machine what the flow angle is, so that velocities can be accurately calculated. Angle correct is further discussed in this chapter (see the section "Review of Doppler Controls").

PW Doppler devices also permit **duplex** imaging where the B-mode image is on the display at the same time as the Doppler signal (Figure 4-35). Duplex imaging allows for real-time adjustment of the Doppler cursor while observing the grayscale image. With duplex imaging, the Doppler and 2D information must be obtained separately. The acquisition of the grayscale information alternates with obtaining the Doppler information. This switching back and forth occurs very fast but does affect the frame rate in a negative way, because it decreases the temporal resolution. **Triplex** imaging is combined grayscale, spectral, and color Doppler information on the screen.

PW Doppler has a major limitation called **aliasing**. Aliasing is a wraparound of the Doppler signal, where the positive shifts are displayed as negative shifts (Figure 4-36). The highest frequency shift that can be measured is equal to one half the **pulse repetition frequency** (PRF), which is known as the **Nyquist limit**. PRF is the number of pulses per second. For example, if the PRF is 2500 Hz, a Doppler shift of 1250 Hz or greater will alias. Aliasing occurs because the Doppler signal must be measured at such a rapid rate. If the PRF is too low, as in the case of a deep blood vessel, the blood cannot be sampled fast enough, and the signal is displayed erroneously (Figure 4-37). In order to eliminate aliasing, either the PRF needs to increase or the Doppler shift needs to decrease. Table 4-20 lists the parameters that can be changed to eliminate aliasing.

In summary, there are certain advantages and disadvantages to both PW and CW Doppler (Table 4-21). The chief advantage of PW Doppler over CW

FIGURE 4-36 Aliasing of the spectral signal. Pulsed-wave Doppler has a major limitation: aliasing. Aliasing is a wraparound of the Doppler signal, where essentially the positive shifts are displayed as negative shifts.

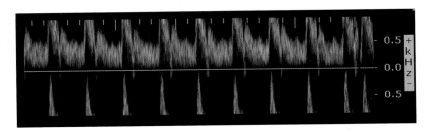

FIGURE 4-37

Explanation of aliasing. When the second hand is observed at 15-second intervals, it appears that the hand is moving in a clockwise direction (**A**). However, when the second hand is observed at 34-second intervals, it appears that the clock is running backwards (**B**). This apparent reversal, or aliasing, is due to not sampling often enough (every 45 seconds instead of every 15 seconds).

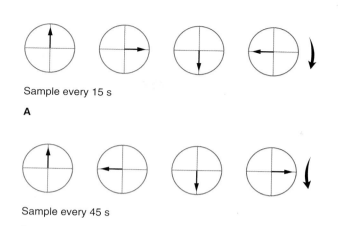

Sample every 15 s

A

Sample every 45 s

B

Doppler is the ability to select a specific depth to sample by utilizing the range gate, thereby offering the user the ability to sample a specific vessel at a specific point. Another advantage of PW Doppler over CW Doppler is the ability to angle correct in order to accurately calculate the velocity of the blood. Though CW Doppler needs two crystals to simultaneously send and receive, the simplest PW Doppler device needs only one crystal to perform this task. However, it must wait for the prior pulse to return before sending the next pulse.

TABLE 4-20 Tools to eliminate aliasing.

Tools to Eliminate Aliasing

- Increase the PRF (scale) setting
- Decrease the sample depth
- Decrease the frequency
- Increase the Doppler angle
- Use continuous-wave transducer

TABLE 4-21 Advantages and disadvantages of continuous-wave Doppler and pulsed-wave Doppler.

Instrument	Advantage	Disadvantage
Continuous-wave Doppler	• High sensitivity • There is no aliasing • Able to measure very high velocities	• Operator cannot select vessel to sample • The signal may have come from any vessel inside the large sample volume
Pulsed-wave Doppler	• Depth of sample volume is operator selectable • User is able to select a specific vessel and sample volume size • Allows for angle correction to accurately measure velocities	• Limited by aliasing • Unable to measure very high velocities

Review of Doppler Controls

Numerous controls are used to manipulate the spectral waveform to aid in diagnosis and interpretation. The range gate, already mentioned in previous sections, is the cursor used in PW Doppler that is placed in the vessel where sampling is desired. The size of the sample volume may be controlled by increasing or decreasing the size of the gate. With CW Doppler, the sampling depth cannot be selected. However, there is a cursor that is placed over the area to be sampled. The sample volume, which is not user controllable with CW Doppler, is larger than PW Doppler and may encompass several blood vessels.

Angle correction is used with PW Doppler in order to more accurately calculate the velocities from the frequency shifts. The "cos θ" portion of the Doppler equation is for the angle correction component (see Table 4-15), in which "θ" is the angle between the Doppler beam and flow. If performing Doppler on a vessel that lies at a 0° angle to the beam, then no angle correction is needed. The 0° angle also provides the most accurate velocity measurements. However, in most clinical practices angles between 30° and 60° are often used. The higher the Doppler angle, the greater the degree of potential error in the measurement. Angles greater than 60° exhibit a very high rate of velocity measurement error, and therefore should be avoided. When using a linear transducer, the Doppler cursor can be steered to either the left or the right. Some machines enable the operator to specify the angle of the steer (e.g., 15° vs. 20°). The advantage of this is that it permits the operator to keep the angle correction at or below 60° by changing the steer angle. In transducers where the steer angle itself cannot be adjusted, the operator may have to "heel" or "toe" the transducer in order to angle correct. The operator must always try to avoid a 90° angle to flow when sampling a vessel (Figure 4-38).

The **scale**, or PRF setting on the machine, is the sampling rate of the Doppler. The sampling rate has to be fast enough in order to accurately plot

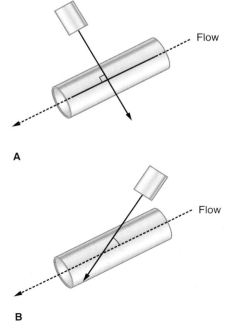

FIGURE 4-38 Proper steering of the Doppler gate. Notice that steering 90° to flow produces an "X," as in "incorrect" (**A**). The correct angle should be equal to or preferably less than 60° (**B**).

the frequency shifts or aliasing will occur. The PRF is determined by the depth. The deeper the vessel, the lower the PRF, and subsequently the higher the risk of aliasing. Likewise, when sampling vessels with high frequency shifts (velocities), the PRF needs to be increased to keep sampling at an adequate rate. If the frequency shift is greater than one half of the PRF (the Nyquist limit) then aliasing will occur. When sampling vessels with slow or hard-to-find flow, the PRF needs to be decreased in order to make the waveform bigger on the screen. A small waveform is poor technique and does not allow for accurate measurements, when needed. Typically, the spectral waveform should occupy two thirds of the spectral display window.

Occasionally, when a deep vessel needs to be imaged the PRF cannot sample at a sufficient rate. Some ultrasound systems solve this dilemma with the use of a high PRF (HPRF) setting, which allows the machine to ignore the **depth ambiguity** problem. When the machine goes into HPRF mode, multiple range gates appear on the screen signifying that the machine is not sure where the pulse is coming from, and could have originated from anywhere along the Doppler cursor.

The **wall filter** is a Doppler control used to eliminate the low-frequency signals caused by wall or heart valve motion. Movement of the heart or vessel walls causes a low-frequency, high-amplitude signal that appears on the spectral display as low-level acoustic **noise**, or **clutter**. Noise takes away from the image and does not contribute useful information and is therefore filtered out with the wall filter. Other names for the wall filter are high-pass and wall-thump filter. In general and vascular imaging, wall motion is not a concern, so the wall filter is kept low. In cardiac imaging, a high wall filter is used to counteract the signal coming from the movement of the myocardium and valves. Caution should be used when applying the wall filter so that useful diastolic information is not removed from the spectral display (Figure 4-39).

The gain of the spectral display can be set independent of the grayscale gain. The brightness of the dots of the spectral display corresponds to the amplitude of the Doppler shift. If the spectral signal is weak, the gain can be increased to improve visualization of the signal. If the spectral gain is too high, it may cause overmeasurement of the spectral waveform, so it is imperative that the gain be set to an appropriate level.

The **baseline**, the movable dividing line between positive and negative frequency shifts, is typically set near the bottom of the spectral display window. However, it should not be set all the way at the bottom of the display or aliasing may be overlooked. Aliasing may be seen if the baseline is too high as well. Lowering the baseline will resolve this problem. Unfortunately, lowering the baseline may eliminate the appearance of aliasing; but, if the Doppler shift is greater than the Nyquist limit, aliasing is still present even if lowering the baseline appears to eliminate the problem (Figure 4-40).

FIGURE 4-39 The use of a wall filter. Notice the absence of diastolic waveform information with the high wall filter.

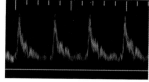
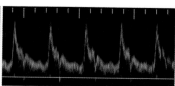

High wall filter   Low wall filter

FIGURE 4-40 Adjusting the baseline. If the baseline is too high (**A**), there appears to be aliasing. Lowering the baseline will eliminate the appearance of aliasing. With the baseline lowered, the aliasing disappears (**B**). Keep in mind that if the frequency shift, 2000 Hz in this case (**B**), is greater than one half the pulse repetition frequency then there is still aliasing, even if you appear to eliminate it by lowering the baseline.

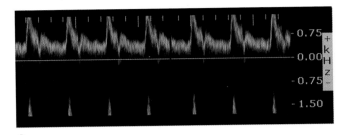

A

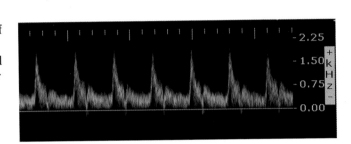

B

Color Doppler Imaging

Color Doppler imaging (CDI), a PW technique, is a color representation of the Doppler shift information superimposed on the grayscale image. CDI provides information pertaining to both the direction and mean velocity of the flow. **Autocorrelation** is the processing technique used to obtain the color flow information, but because it is relatively fast, it is not as accurate as FFT. CDI only provides the mean velocity information and not maximum velocities.

CDI also uses a larger gate than spectral Doppler, a gate that is made up of many scan lines proportional to the width of the gate. Color information is obtained at many points along each scan line and each pulse packet is checked for movement, opposed to nonmovement, by searching for frequency shifts. Moving reflectors are specified as a color and nonmoving reflectors are specified as a shade of gray.

The **ensemble length**, also known as the **packet size**, is the number of pulses per scan line within the color gate. The higher the ensemble length, the more sampling points along each scan line, and therefore, the higher the sensitivity of the color signal. High ensemble lengths increase the ability to detect slow flow and offer a more accurate mean velocity. Unfortunately, this is at the expense of the frame rate, which is very low with high ensemble lengths. The ensemble length can be as low as 3 pulses per scan line but is typically around 10 to 20 pulses per scan line. Another disadvantage of high ensemble lengths is the machine's inability to detect rapidly changing hemodynamic events secondary to the longer acquisition time. CDI is slow, and large gates and/or high ensemble lengths slow it down even further. For the best frame rate, the smallest color gate should always be employed (Table 4-22).

The color Doppler scale shows direction of flow as a color or range of colors on each side of a black baseline (Figure 4-41). Black within a color display means that either there was no Doppler shift present in that location

TABLE 4-22 Ensemble length and color Doppler.
Results of Higher Ensemble Lengths
• More pulses per scan line
• More sensitive to slow flow
• More accurate mean velocity
• Slower frame rate (temporal resolution)

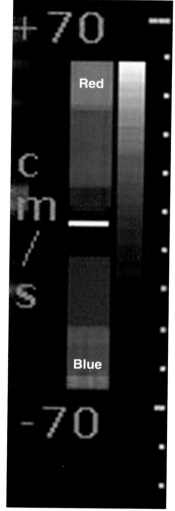

FIGURE 4-41 The color Doppler scale. Typically, flow toward the transducer is displayed in red or above the baseline (*white line separating colors*), while flow away from the transducer is displayed in blue or below the baseline. A color version of this figure can be found on thePoint. Refer to the inside front cover for log-in instructions.

(as a result of either a 90° angle to flow or no flow), or the shift was so low that it was eliminated by wall filters. In general and vascular imaging, the color scale is often set by convention, so that red represents arteries and blue represents veins. In cardiac imaging, the color scale is thought of as **BART**: blue away, red toward. However, the color scale can be inverted, so that blue is toward and red is away.

The color scale is most commonly presented in **velocity mode**, where the colors are vertically oriented for positive/negative shifts. Another mode, associated with cardiac imaging, is **variance mode**, where colors are represented vertically and shades of green are oriented horizontally to denote the presence of turbulence. There are three main components of the color imaging: **hue**, **saturation**, and **brightness** (or **luminance**).

The hue of a color is the color itself as determined by its wavelength. A color can be made to appear lighter by adding white to it. Saturation is how much white is added compared to the original color. The less white in the color, the more saturated it is. Pink, for example, is less saturated than red. The brightness of the color is how intense the color is and related to the amplitude of the signal.One of the more challenging aspects of CDI is identifying direction of color flow just by looking at the image and the color scale (Figure 4-42).

Color Aliasing

As a PW technique, CDI is bound by the same limitation as PW spectral Doppler. Therefore, aliasing can occur. Aliasing on CDI is represented by a wraparound of the color scale (Figure 4-43). As with spectral Doppler, aliasing can be eliminated by increasing the PRF/scale. Appropriate setting of the color PRF allows for setting the proper sensitivity to flow. Low PRF color settings are used for slow or difficult-to-demonstrate flow, and high PRF settings are used for fast flow and also to eliminate aliasing. In addition to PRF, color Doppler also has a gain setting, and it is imperative that the gain is set properly. If the color gain is set too high, the result is color noise throughout the color gate. If the color gain is set too low, the vessel will not be adequately filled with color.

In the presence of very slow flow, or if small vessels are being analyzed, it may be helpful to average multiple frames instead of displaying only one frame of color information at a time. Increasing the **persistence** setting reduces the effect of noise and makes it easier to follow small vessels. The trade-off of high persistence is a decrease in the frame rate.

When both grayscale and color information are present within the same pixel, **color priority** is a setting on the machine that allows the operator to set a threshold for displaying color pixels instead of grayscale pixels.

FIGURE 4-42 How to determine the direction of flow. Draw a line from the overhanging corner of the Doppler gate. Call this "the transducer" for the sake of this demonstration. Notice how the blood flow in this vessel is red. Look at the color scale: red is "away from the transducer." Therefore, flow is moving in a direction away from the line that represents the transducer, or toward the left of the screen. A color version of this figure can be found on thePoint. Refer to the inside front cover for log-in instructions.

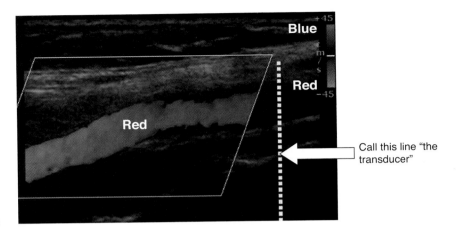

A pixel, the smallest component of an ultrasound image, can either be a color or shade of gray, not both at the same time. Priority sets the threshold that the amplitude (i.e., brightness of the shade of gray) will have to exceed in order for grayscale pixels to be displayed rather than color pixels. Below that threshold, color pixels will be placed. If the priority is set too low, then image noise or artifacts within the vessel will be displayed instead of color pixels. A higher priority setting is useful in filling a vessel with color when there is a low signal-to-noise ratio.

Tissue Doppler Imaging

Specifically used for cardiac imaging, **tissue Doppler imaging (TDI)** is another CDI technique. Flowing blood typically produces a low-amplitude, high-velocity signal. However, myocardial wall motion produces a high-amplitude, low-velocity signal. Instead of using a high-pass filter to filter out the signal from the wall motion, TDI uses a low-passfilter to eliminate the signal from the blood and only show color information representing the wall motion. TDI is still limited by frequency shifts at 90° angles; but since the myocardial walls are oriented 0° to the beam in some views, this is not a limitation. TDI can be performed with color Doppler and spectral Doppler display modes.

FIGURE 4-43 Color Doppler aliasing. Aliasing on color Doppler imaging is represented by a wraparound of the color scale. A color version of this figure can be found on thePoint. Refer to the inside front cover for log-in instructions.

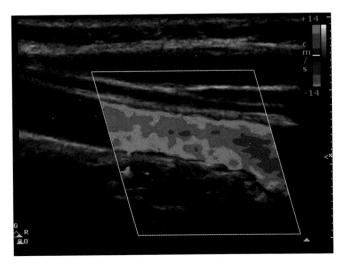
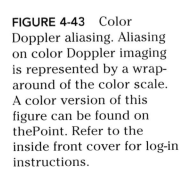

Power Doppler

PW spectral and color Doppler are limited by flow at 90° angles, because the frequency shift on which the flow information is based is equal to 0 at that critical angle. **Power Doppler**, also termed color Doppler energy or power angio, ignores the frequency shift information and focuses only on the amplitude, or strength, of the shift. Power Doppler is only able to display amplitude information and does not provide information on velocity or direction of flow. Power Doppler is almost completely independent of angle, which makes it quite functional for evaluating slow flowing and/or tortuous vessels. Both an advantage and a disadvantage of power Doppler is its sensitivity. Since power Doppler is very sensitive, it is ideal for slow, small vessels, but it also makes it more susceptible to patient or organ motion. **Flash artifact** occurs when power Doppler is being used and inadvertent motion interrupts the quality of the signal.

Directional Power Doppler

A relatively new technique called **directional power Doppler** was created to compensate for the disadvantages of color and power Doppler. With directional power Doppler, power Doppler (amplitude) information is displayed on top of color (directional) flow information to produce a composite image.

Doppler Artifacts

There are several Doppler artifacts. Table 4-23 provides an explanation of them.

T A B L E 4 - 2 3 Doppler artifacts, their definitions, and means to fix the image.		
Artifact	**Definition**	**Quick Fix**
Clutter	Acoustic noise eliminated with high-pass wall filters	Increase wall filter
Aliasing	Pulsed-wave artifact caused by insufficient sampling of flow	Increase PRF, decrease frequency shift, or use CW
Mirror image	Reproduction of spectral or color information opposite a strong reflector	Decrease gain or angle (must be <90°)
Blooming	Overgained color or spectral waveform causing signal to be larger than it should be	Decrease gain or transmit power
High PRF (depth ambiguity)	HPRF setting in PW Doppler means the PW is emulating a CW probe and is unsure of where echoes came from	Change depth or Doppler angle
Flash artifact	Excessive color signal in surrounding tissue caused by movement during power Doppler	Decrease gain or increase PRF. If possible, eliminate source of motion (e.g., with a breath hold)

REVIEW QUESTIONS

1. What provides the potential energy in the cardiovascular system?
   a. Distal arterioles
   b. Blood flowing through the vessels
   c. Beating heart
   d. Venous system

2. What is another term for gravitational potential energy?
   a. Kinetic energy
   b. Viscous energy
   c. Inertial energy
   d. Hydrostatic pressure

3. What is the name of the flat flow profile that is seen at the entrance of vessels?
   a. Plug flow
   b. Laminar flow
   c. Turbulent flow
   d. Chaotic flow

4. What does increasing the PRF/scale setting on a spectral Doppler do?
   a. Increases the potential of aliasing
   b. Decreases the potential of aliasing
   c. Makes the spectral waveform appear larger
   d. Optimizes the system to detect slow flow

5. Which of the following is seen with continuous-wave instrumentation?
   a. Transducer frequency matches that of the oscillator
   b. Sample depth can be determined by a range gate
   c. Very short pulses are used
   d. Aliasing limits velocity measurements

6. When is the Doppler shift highest?
   a. Doppler shift is unrelated to beam angle
   b. When the beam is perpendicular to the direction of flow
   c. When the beam is parallel to the direction of flow
   d. When the beam is at a 45° angle to flow

7. Which of the following will **not** eliminate aliasing?
   a. Increasing the PRF
   b. Increasing the Nyquist limit above the frequency shift
   c. Decreasing the sample depth
   d. Increasing the frequency shift above the Nyquist limit

8. When a reflector moves toward the transducer, what will happen to the reflected frequency?
   a. Increase
   b. Decrease
   c. Stay the same
   d. It is not possible to predict

9. Which of the following has to be increased in order to see an increase in flow volume?
   a. Pressure difference
   b. Resistance
   c. Vessel length
   d. Viscosity

10. Adjusting which of the following will have no effect on the measured frequency shift?
    a. Flow velocity
    b. Operating frequency
    c. Amplitude
    d. Propagation speed

11. Which of the following is representative of Ohm's law?
    a. $V = IR$
    b. $I = R/V$
    c. $R = I/V$
    d. $R = VI$

12. What is the point at which Reynolds number predicts turbulence?
    a. 500
    b. 1200
    c. 2000
    d. 4000

13. In order to maintain flow as a constant, if the area of a vessel increases what must happen to the velocity?
    a. It increases
    b. It decreases
    c. It does not change with changes in area
    d. Not enough information

14. Which of the following is **not** a way in which venous blood is assisted in returning to the heart?
    a. Calf muscle pump
    b. Inspiration
    c. Expiration
    d. Venous valves

15. In a standing patient, where is the hydrostatic pressure the highest?
    a. In the feet
    b. In the arms
    c. In the abdomen
    d. Near the heart

16. A stenosis of 75% in area is equal to what percent of stenosis in diameter?
    a. 25%
    b. 50%
    c. 75%
    d. 100%

17. In the exercising patient, what is the response to peripheral resistance with arteriolar dilatation?
    a. The peripheral resistance increases
    b. The peripheral resistance decreases
    c. There is no change in peripheral resistance
    d. Peripheral resistance would decrease but only in presence of disease

18. Which of the following will be seen with a stationary reflector?
    a. There is a higher reflected frequency compared with the incident frequency
    b. There is a lower reflected frequency compared with the incident frequency

c. The incident frequency is equal to the reflected frequency
d. The reflected intensity is higher than the incident intensity

19. What happens as the frequency of the transducer increases?
    a. Penetration ability is increased
    b. The amount of scatter is increased
    c. The frequency shift is decreased
    d. The amount of attenuation is decreased

20. What occurs as the Doppler angle is increased?
    a. It decreases the frequency shift
    b. It increases the frequency shift
    c. It increases the risk for aliasing
    d. It improves the accuracy of the velocity calculation

21. What is the component of the ultrasound machine used to detect positive versus negative frequency shifts?
    a. Analog Doppler
    b. Oscillator
    c. Fourier transformer
    d. Phase quadrature

22. Which of the following is true for continuous-wave Doppler devices?
    a. It only needs to have one piezoelectric element
    b. It must have at least two piezoelectric elements
    c. It must have three piezoelectric elements
    d. No piezoelectric elements are needed for CW Doppler

23. Which of the following will result in aliasing?
    a. Too low an operating frequency
    b. Increased sampling of the blood flow
    c. Undersampling of the blood flow
    d. Too high a Doppler angle

24. Which mathematical processing technique is used to analyze the data and produce a spectral waveform?
    a. Amplitude shifting
    b. Autocorrelation
    c. Amplitude sampling
    d. Fast Fourier transform

25. Which of the following represents the resistive index?
    a. Peak systolic velocity minus the end diastolic velocity divided by the mean velocity
    b. End diastolic velocity minus the peak systolic velocity divided by the peak systolic velocity
    c. Peak systolic velocity minus the end diastolic velocity divided by the peak systolic velocity
    d. Peak systolic velocity minus the end diastolic velocity divided by the end diastolic velocity

26. What does the brightness of the dots that make up the spectral display represent?
    a. The number of red blood cells present
    b. The velocity of the signal
    c. The frequency shift
    d. The amount of turbulence present

27. What is said to occur when the window of the spectral Doppler display is filled-in?
    a. There is spectral broadening
    b. There is laminar flow
    c. The Doppler gate is small and centered within the vessel
    d. There is only one velocity at a given point in time

28. In order to add more spectral Doppler waveforms to the display, what setting on the machine should be adjusted?
    a. PRF
    b. Sweep speed
    c. Heart rate
    d. Gain

29. Which of the following may result if the spectral Doppler gain is too high?
    a. Too much output power sent into the patient
    b. Undermeasurement of the velocities
    c. Overmeasurement of the velocities
    d. An image that is too dark

30. The Doppler shift is lowest at what angle to flow?
    a. 0°
    b. 45°
    c. 60°
    d. 90°

31. Which signal processing technique used for color Doppler is not as accurate, but faster, than the technique used for spectral Doppler?
    a. Zero crossing
    b. Phase quadrature
    c. Autocorrelation
    d. Fast Fourier transform

32. What is the fewest number of crystals a PW Doppler device may have?
    a. Zero
    b. One
    c. Two
    d. Three

33. Which type of Doppler does not rely on the frequency shift but instead relies on the strength of the shift?
    a. Spectral Doppler
    b. Power Doppler
    c. Color Doppler imaging
    d. CW Doppler

34. What is it called when the 2D image, color Doppler image, and spectral Doppler are displayed simultaneously?
    a. Duplex mode
    b. Triplex mode
    c. Phase quadrature mode
    d. Multiplex mode

35. What is the duty factor of CW Doppler?
    a. 1
    b. 100
    c. 0.01
    d. 1%

36. Which of the following is true about CW Doppler?
    a. The measured frequency shifts come from a user-selected depth
    b. A range gate is placed in the vessel to be sampled
    c. There is a large sample volume that obtains signals from all vessels within
    d. Pulses of sound are sent into the tissue to measure the frequency shifts

37. When compared to 2D grayscale imaging, which of the following color Doppler statements is true?
    a. There is improved temporal resolution
    b. There is worse temporal resolution
    c. There are fewer pulses per scan line
    d. There is a higher frame rate

38. Which of the following statements is false?
    a. Aliasing does not occur with color Doppler
    b. Continuous-wave Doppler is able to measure very high frequency shifts
    c. Pulsed-wave Doppler has range resolution
    d. Power Doppler is not limited by 90° angle

39. Which of the following frequency shifts would exhibit aliasing if the PRF is 5000 Hz?
    a. 1.0 kHz
    b. 2.5 kHz
    c. 3.0 kHz
    d. None of the above

40. Which of the following is true about the frequency shift?
    a. It increases with an increase in Doppler angle
    b. It is typically greater than 20,000 Hz
    c. It is inversely related to operating frequency
    d. It is in the audible range of sound

41. What can be said about the ensemble length of pulsed-wave Doppler?
    a. It is less than 3 pulses per scan line
    b. It is more than 100 pulses per scan line
    c. It is about 10 to 20 pulses per scan line
    d. It is typically 0

42. What happens if blood flow is sampled in the center of laminar flow?
    a. There will be a higher velocity than if sampled toward the edges
    b. There will be a slower velocity than if sampled toward the edges
    c. It will be made up of many different velocities
    d. It will be turbulent

43. Which of the following is false about color Doppler imaging?
    a. It is prone to aliasing
    b. It obtains mean velocity information
    c. It uses autocorrelation as its signal processing technique
    d. It can measure peak systolic and end diastolic velocities

44. Which of the following is a property of power Doppler?
    a. Able to obtain velocity information and direction of flow
    b. Signal is obtained by detecting amplitude of shift
    c. It is prone to aliasing
    d. Limited by perpendicular angle of incidence

45. Assuming flow is constant, what happens in a region of blood vessel narrowing?
    a. There is a significant pressure increase
    b. There is an increase in the velocity along with a corresponding increase in pressure
    c. There is an increase in the velocity along with a corresponding decrease in pressure
    d. Velocity and pressure are unchanged

46. Which of the following is true about the spectral Doppler envelope?
    a. It is thin when there are many different velocities
    b. It is thin with CW Doppler
    c. It is thickened in the center of a laminar flow vessel
    d. It is thickened in the presence of turbulence

47. What is the term for the pressure difference between the inside of a vein and the tissue outside?
    a. Hydrostatic pressure
    b. Autocorrelation
    c. Transmural pressure
    d. Kinetic energy

48. A proximal stenosis will look like what on the spectral waveform?
    a. Reversal of flow in diastole
    b. Delay in the systolic upstroke
    c. Triphasic waveform
    d. Aliasing

49. The end diastolic component is missing on a spectral waveform. Which of the following should be adjusted to fix this?
    a. Gain
    b. Scale
    c. Wall filter
    d. Frequency

50. In the exercising patient, the distal arterioles are dilated. What type of flow pattern would most likely be demonstrated on spectral Doppler within the proximal vessels?
    a. Monophasic
    b. Biphasic
    c. Triphasic
    d. Venous

SUGGESTED READINGS

Belloni FL. Teaching the principles of hemodynamics. Adv Physiol Educ 1999;22(1):S187–S202.

Daigle RJ. Techniques in Non-Invasive Vascular Diagnosis. 3rd Ed. Littleton, CO: Summer Publishing, 2008.

Edelman SK. Understanding Ultrasound Physics. 3rd Ed. Woodlands, TX: ESP Inc., 2005.

Fox TF. Arterial hemodynamics for the vascular sonographer. Vascular Ultrasound Today 2008;8(13):159–176.

Hedrick WR, Hykes DL, Starchman DE. Ultrasound Physics and Instrumentation. 4th Ed. St. Louis, MO: Mosby, 2005.

Kremkau FW. Diagnostic Ultrasound: Principles and Instruments. 7th Ed. St. Louis, MO: Saunders, 2006.

Miele FR. Ultrasound Physics and Instrumentation. 4th Ed. Forney, TX: Miele Enterprises, 2006.

Milnor WR. Hemodynamics. 2nd Ed. Baltimore, MD: Williams & Wilkins, 1989.

Oh JK, Seward TB, Tajik AJ. The Echo Manual. Lippincott Williams & Wilkins, 2007.

Rumwell C, McPharlin M. Vascular Technology: An Illustrated Review. 4th Ed. Pasadena, CA: Davies, 2009.

Strandness DE. Duplex Scanning in Vascular Disorders. 3rd Ed. Philadelphia, PA: Lippincott Williams & Wilkins, 2002.

Taylor KJ, Burns PN, Wells NT. Clinical Applications of Doppler Ultrasound. New York, NY: Raven Press, 1988.

Thrush A, Hartshorne T. Vascular Ultrasound: How, Why, and When. 3rd Ed. London: Elsevier, 2009.

Zwiebel W, Pellerito J. Introduction to Vascular Sonography. 5th Ed. Philadelphia, PA: Elsevier, 2005.

CHAPTER 5

Quality Assurance

INTRODUCTION

A quality assurance program in the ultrasound department is critical to system accuracy and patient care. It must be completed on a routine schedule. Preventative maintenance may be performed semiannually or annually. Several testing phantoms exist to ensure correct equipment operation. The primary objective for completing quality assurance is the confirmation that image quality is optimal and that subtle changes in function are detected.

KEY TERMS

AIUM test object—an outdated test object that used an acrylic tank filled with fluid; the fluid in this test object attempted to simulate the speed of sound in soft tissue

axial resolution—the ability to accurately identify reflectors that are arranged parallel to the ultrasound beam

contrast resolution—the ability to differentiate one shade of gray from another

Doppler phantom—the test object used to evaluate the flow direction, the depth capability or penetration of the Doppler beam, and the accuracy of the sample volume location and measured velocity

elevational resolution—the resolution in the third dimension of the beam: the slice-thickness plane

grayscale test objects—the testing phantoms that allow the evaluation of an ultrasound machine's ability to test grayscale sensitivity (contrast resolution) using various transducer frequencies

horizontal calibration—the ability to place echoes in the proper location horizontally and perpendicular to the sound beam

lab accreditation—a voluntary process that acknowledges an organization's competency and credibility according to standards and essentials set forth by a reliable source

lateral resolution—the ability to accurately identify reflectors that are arranged perpendicular to the ultrasound beam

preventative maintenance—a methodical way of evaluating equipment's performance on a routine basis to ensure proper and accurate equipment function

quality assurance program—a planned program consisting of scheduled equipment-testing activities that confirm correct performance of equipment

registration—the ability to place echoes in the correct location

sample volume—the area within the range gate where the Doppler signals are obtained

sensitivity—the ability of a system to display low-level or weak echoes

slice-thickness phantom—the test object that evaluates the elevational resolution, or the thickness portion, of the sound beam perpendicular to the imaging plane

tissue-equivalent phantom—the test object that mimics the acoustic properties of human tissue and is used to ensure proper equipment performance
vertical depth—the distance from the transducer

PREVENTATIVE MAINTENANCE

An ultrasound department should have a well-planned and formatted **preventative maintenance** program for every piece of imaging equipment in the sonography lab. Every transducer and machine must be evaluated. The American Institute of Ultrasound in Medicine (AIUM) suggests that all ultrasound equipment should be kept in good working order and be evaluated and calibrated annually. Routine electrical evaluation should be done by a sonographer to ensure that electrical cords are intact and do not present an electrical hazard to both the sonographer and the patient. Routine cleaning of the machine's vents and outer surfaces should be performed to assure that the equipment is in optimal working condition. The machine should be completely wiped down with an approved disinfectant before and after completing portable ultrasound procedures. The prevention of the spread of infection is further discussed in Chapter 6.

A record of each inspection, evaluation, and calibration must be maintained in the ultrasound department. When a sonographer notices that a transducer or equipment is out of calibration or producing nondiagnostic images, the service engineer must be contacted to evaluate the equipment. The equipment should not be used until the service engineer has corrected the problem. The sonographer is also responsible for maintaining a comprehensive **quality assurance program** for the department. Accrediting agencies publish specific guidelines identifying standards for quality assurance in the ultrasound lab.

EQUIPMENT MALFUNCTION AND TROUBLESHOOTING

All equipment malfunctions should be reported immediately. If a problem is identified that may be a potential hazard for the sonographer or the patient, the machine should be pulled from operation and stored until an engineer can assess the status of the equipment. For example, frayed cords or cracked transducer housing could be a potential electrical hazard for both the sonographer and the patient.

Most manufacturers have technical support that can troubleshoot the problem via the telephone. The machine's owners manual may also be helpful in troubleshooting minor problems or assisting in the correct operation of an equipment feature. More complicated malfunctions require the on-site evaluation of the equipment by a service engineer.

PERFORMANCE TESTING

Daily operation should be observed by the sonographer and errors or concerns reported immediately. Daily operation characteristics may include evaluating the electrical cords and transducer cords for fraying or tears in the wire casing, evaluating the face of the transducer for cracks or chips, evaluating for nonfunctioning or sticking keys on the keyboard, evaluating for a non-mobile trackball, and evaluating for obvious caliper malfunctions, irregular technique, or depth adjustments.

Detailed and specific performance testing should be completed on a routinely scheduled basis, because gradual degradation of the sonographic image may be difficult to detect. Performance testing includes scheduled activities that evaluate the accuracy of the system's imaging capabilities (Table 5-1). Imaging capabilities include **axial resolution** and **lateral resolution**, **vertical depth** and **horizontal calibration**, and overall **registration** of data. If the image appears to be nonrepresentative of the anatomy, or the transducer appears to have a bad element or functions erratically, then service should be scheduled immediately and the machine or transducer taken out of service.

T A B L E 5 - 1 Imaging properties.

Imaging Property	Description	Interpretation
Axial resolution	The ability to accurately identify reflectors that are arranged parallel to the ultrasound beam	Correct placement and measurement of the reflectors indicate that the spatial pulse length is consistent with manufacturer's requirements.
Lateral resolution	The ability to accurately identify reflectors that are arranged perpendicular to the ultrasound beam	Correct placement and measurement of the reflectors indicate that the beam former and transducer's elements are working correctly.
Dead zone	Tests the ability of reflectors to be accurately imaged within the first centimeter of the sound beam as it leaves the transducer's face	When the dead zone area shifts deeper, then the pulsing of the system or a transducer element may be compromised.
Registration	The ability to accurately identify a pin with accuracy in size and location (vertical distance and horizontal distance) Note: Range accuracy is also called vertical depth calibration	Accuracy of measurement is vital to the successful diagnostic capabilities of an imaging system. Each vertical and horizontal pin must be accurately represented in size and location.
Sensitivity and uniformity	The ability of the system to detect echoes (including weak echoes) and display them uniformly with the same brightness on the monitor	Transducer failure or output variations can cause loss of echo sensitivity and image uniformity. With the correct time gain compensation, similar reflectors should appear on the monitor as the same, regardless of their depth.

Test objects, or phantoms, are used to accurately calibrate ultrasound imaging equipment. Test objects include calibration test objects, tissue-mimicking test objects, and Doppler test objects (**Doppler phantoms**). Each test object has a specific purpose and may have one or more imaging parameters that it is capable of evaluating. Calibration test objects evaluate the measurement accuracy of the machine. The tissue-mimicking test objects, or **grayscale test objects**, are used to evaluate a machine's grayscale **sensitivity** and **contrast resolution**, at varying frequencies and depths. Sensitivity is the machine's ability to detect very weak echoes. Contrast resolution is the ability to differentiate one shade of gray from another. Tissue-mimicking test objects are often combined with calibration test objects to create a general-purpose phantom.

Doppler test objects are used to evaluate the flow direction, the depth capability or penetration of the Doppler beam, and the accuracy of **sample volume** location and measured velocity. Each phantom is supplied with testing directions and interpretation results. Detailed records should be kept in a log with each transducer and imaging system. Any variances over the recommended allowance must be reported and investigated by a service engineer. A detailed log of every service call or malfunction should be maintained for each imaging system. The next section describes the different phantoms that may be used to test and calibrate the ultrasound machine.

AIUM 100 mm Test Object

The AIUM 100 mm test object is no longer used for quality assurance since the advent of the **tissue-equivalent phantom** (Figure 5-1). However, this test object's construction and usefulness are still vital to understand. The **AIUM test object** was an acrylic tank that was filled with fluid. The fluid in this tank attempted to simulate the speed of sound in soft tissue. Attenuation properties of soft tissue were not simulated. Inside the tank, there were several stainless steel pins that represented various performance characteristics of an imaging system. The AIUM test object was designed to allow imaging from each side.

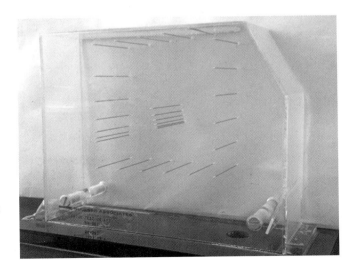

FIGURE 5-1 The American Institute of Ultrasound in Medicine (AIUM) 100 mm test object.

Tissue-Equivalent Phantom

A tissue-equivalent, or tissue-mimicking, phantom is a test object used to test the accuracy and grayscale imaging of ultrasound imaging systems (Figure 5-2). The phantom, which is made up of an aqueous gel and graphite particles, transmits sound at 1540 m/s and attenuates at a rate similar to that of soft tissue. Stainless steel pins are strategically located throughout the phantom so that accurate identification and location can be recorded. Structures mimicking cysts and solid masses are also positioned in the phantom (Figures 5-3 and 5-4).

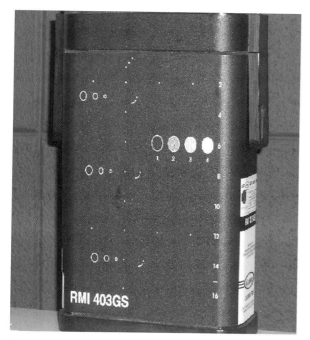

FIGURE 5-2   The tissue-equivalent phantom.

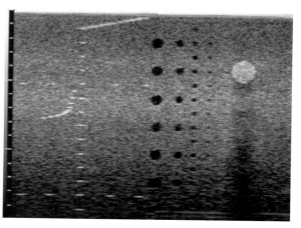

FIGURE 5-3   The sonographic appearance of the tissue-equivalent phantom. (Courtesy ATS Laboratories.)

Model 539 Multipurpose Phantom
ATS Laboratories, Incorporated, Bridgeport, CT, USA

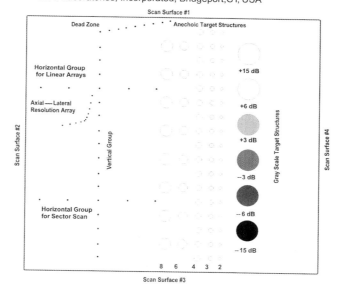

FIGURE 5-4   The anatomy of the tissue-equivalent phantom. (Courtesy ATS Laboratories.)

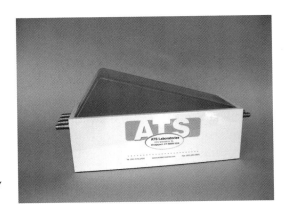

FIGURE 5-5 A Doppler testing phantom. (Courtesy ATS Laboratories.)

The tissue-equivalent phantom's integrity must be maintained, as the container must be airtight to avoid degradation of the tissue properties inside the phantom. Also, the storage area temperature should also be monitored to preserve the acoustic properties of the phantom. Sonographers should always check the manufacturer's instructions on proper care and maintenance for the phantom.

Doppler Testing Phantom

The Doppler testing phantom evaluates the Doppler capabilities of imaging systems. These phantoms utilize a physical moving structure, such as a vibrating string, a moving belt, or a circulation pump that moves blood-simulating fluid through the phantom. Thus, Doppler sensitivity, depth resolution, volume flow, and velocity accuracy can all be evaluated using a Doppler phantom (Figure 5-5).

Slice-Thickness Phantom

A **slice-thickness phantom** evaluates the **elevational resolution**, or the thickness portion, of the sound beam perpendicular to the imaging plane. In the event that the sound beam is too thick, echoes appear inside cystic or fluid-filled structures (Figures 5-6 and 5-7).

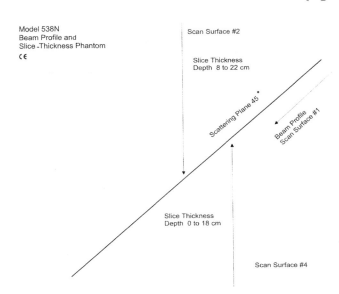

FIGURE 5-6 The anatomy of the slice-thickness phantom. (Courtesy ATS Laboratories.)

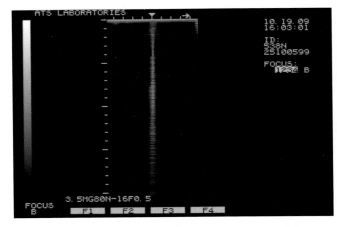

FIGURE 5-7 The sonographic appearance of the slice-thickness phantom. (Courtesy ATS Laboratories.)

LAB ACCREDITATION AND CREDENTIALING

Reputable organizations exist that recognize ultrasound labs for their compliance with national performance standards. **Lab accreditation** procedures mandate that the lab should meet specific, comprehensive guidelines governing departmental administration and policies, patient care, scanning protocols, and procedures.

Accrediting Agencies

Accrediting agencies in the field of sonography include the AIUM, Intersocietal Commission for the Accreditation of Vascular Laboratories (ICAVL), Intersocietal Commission for the Accreditation of Echocardiography Laboratories (ICAEL), and American College of Radiology (ACR). The AIUM is an organization that accredits ultrasound labs in the abdominal, small parts, gynecology and obstetrics, and vascular modalities. ICAVL offers accreditation for vascular labs throughout the world. ICAEL provides peer-reviewed echocardiography laboratory accreditation. The ACR also provides opportunity for volunteer accreditation for radiology-based ultrasound labs. Each of these agencies plays a vital role in maintaining the standards of care that our patients both expect and deserve (Table 5-2).

Professional Credentialing

Professional credentialing of sonographers and interpreting physicians is recommended for health care professionals practicing sonographic procedures. Lab accrediting organizations require professional certification(s) for practicing sonographers. Currently, three credentialing organizations exist: the American Registry of Diagnostic Medical Sonography (ARDMS), Cardiovascular Credential International (CCI), and the American Registry of Radiographic Technologists (ARRT).

The ARDMS represents thousands of certified sonographers throughout the world. Certification exams are offered in several modalities. CCI offers certification exams in cardiac and vascular testing. The ARRT offers multiple certification exams in diagnostic imaging, with a specialty in sonography (Table 5-3).

TABLE 5-2 Accrediting agencies and their Web sites.

Accrediting Agency	Web Site
American College of Radiology (ACR)	http://www.acr.org/
American Institute of Ultrasound in Medicine (AIUM)	http://www.aium.org/
Intersocietal Commission for the Accreditation of Echocardiography Laboratories (ICAEL)	http://www.icael.org/icael/index.htm
Intersocietal Commission for the Accreditation of Vascular Laboratories (ICAVL)	http://www.icavl.org/icavl/index.htm

T A B L E **5 - 3** Credential granting organizations and their Web sites.	
Credential Granting Organization	**Web Site**
American Registry of Diagnostic Medical Sonography (ARDMS)	http://www.ardms.org
American Registry of Radiographic Technologists (ARRT)	https://www.arrt.org/
Cardiovascular Credential International (CCI)	http://www.cci-online.org/

REVIEW QUESTIONS

1. Comprehensive preventative maintenance must be performed at least:
   a. Daily
   b. Semiannually
   c. Annually
   d. When a problem occurs

2 Which test object uses a moving belt, vibrating string or a fluid pump?
   a. AIUM phantom
   b. tissue-mimicking phantom
   c. slice-thickness phantom
   d. Doppler phantom

3. The AIUM test object can evaluate all of the following except:
   a. Vertical distance
   b. Horizontal distance
   c. Contrast resolution
   d. Axial resolution

4. The test used to evaluate the depth of reflectors from a transducer is called:
   a. Horizontal depth calibration
   b. Vertical depth calibration
   c. Dead zone
   d. Lateral resolution

5. All of the following are goals for a quality assurance program except:
   a. Document proper equipment performance
   b. Optimize image quality consistently
   c. Keep detailed results from quality assurance testing
   d. Report equipment malfunctions annually

6. The only certifying agency that offers credentialing exams for cardiac and vascular testing is:
   a. ACR
   b. AIUM
   c. ICAVL
   d. CCI

7. Which of the following is a voluntary process that acknowledges an organization's competency and credibility according to standards and essentials set forth by a reliable source?
   a. Credentialing
   b. Accreditation

    c. Licensure
    d. Registration

8. Which of the following is the system's ability to detect weak echoes?
    a. Uniformity
    b. Registration
    c. Sensitivity
    d. Dead zone

9. What type of errors will cause artificial echoes to appear within a cystic structure?
    a. Dead zone
    b. Registration
    c. Slice thickness
    d. Contrast resolution

10. Which of the following indicates the maximum depth of visualization?
    a. Vertical distance
    b. Horizontal distance
    c. Lateral resolution
    d. Sensitivity

11. Which of the following is a methodical way of evaluating equipment's performance on a routine basis to ensure proper and accurate equipment function?
    a. Accreditation
    b. Quality assurance
    c. Preventative maintenance
    d. Credentialing

12. Who among the following is responsible for ensuring an effective quality assurance program in the sonography lab?
    a. Physician
    b. Engineer
    c. Biomedical specialist
    d. Sonographer

13. Which of the following is the ability to accurately identify reflectors that are arranged front to back and parallel to the ultrasound beam?
    a. Registration
    b. Vertical distance
    c. Axial resolution
    d. Lateral resolution

14. Which of the following test phantoms should be stored in an airtight container and in a controlled temperature?
    a. AIUM test object
    b. Doppler testing phantom
    c. Tissue-equivalent phantom
    d. String phantom

15. Which of the following is the test object that evaluates the elevation resolution, or the thickness portion, of the sound beam perpendicular to the imaging plane?
    a. AIUM test object
    b. Doppler testing phantom
    c. Tissue-equivalent phantom
    d. Slice-thickness phantom

16. Which of the following is an outdated test object that used an acrylic tank filled with fluid that attempted to simulate the speed of sound in soft tissue?
    a. AIUM test object
    b. Doppler testing phantom
    c. Tissue-equivalent phantom
    d. Slice-thickness phantom

17. The test object that mimics the acoustic properties of human tissue and is used to ensure proper equipment performance is:
    a. AIUM test object
    b. Doppler testing phantom
    c. Tissue-equivalent phantom
    d. Slice-thickness phantom

18. Which of the following does the Doppler phantom not typically evaluate?
    a. Flow direction
    b. Subtle tissue differences
    c. Depth capability of the beam
    d. Accuracy of sample volume location

19. Which of the following is not an accrediting agency of sonography labs?
    a. American Institute of Ultrasound in Medicine
    b. American Registry of Diagnostic Medical Sonography
    c. Intersocietal Commission for the Accreditation of Vascular Laboratories
    d. American College of Radiology

20. Which of the following is not a credential granting body for sonographers?
    a. American Registry of Diagnostic Medical Sonography
    b. Cardiovascular Credential International
    c. American Registry of Radiographic Technologists
    d. American Institute of Ultrasound in Medicine

SUGGESTED READINGS

Edelman SK. Understanding Ultrasound Physics. 3rd Ed. Woodlands, TX: ESP Inc., 2005.

Hedrick WR, Hykes DL, Starchman DE. Ultrasound Physics and Instrumentation. 4th Ed. St. Louis, MO: Mosby, 2005.

Kremkau FW. Diagnostic Ultrasound: Principles and Instruments. 7th Ed. St. Louis, MO: Saunders, 2006.

Zagzebski JA. Essentials of Ultrasound Physics. St. Louis, MO: Mosby, 1996.

CHAPTER 6

Patient Care

INTRODUCTION

This brief chapter will be used to discuss the role of the sonographer in patient care and the possible bioeffects of diagnostic ultrasound. Infection control and the practice of universal precautions will be stressed as well.

KEY TERMS

acoustic cavitation–the production of bubbles in a liquid medium

automatic external defibrillator–a portable device that is used to detect and treat abnormal heart rhythms with electrical defibrillation

diabetes mellitus–a group of metabolic diseases that result from a chronic disorder of carbohydrate metabolism

diabetic ketoacidosis–a complication of diabetes that results from a severe lack of insulin

Health Insurance Portability and Accountability Act–the Act enacted in 1996 by the United States Congress, which, among many goals, upholds patient confidentiality and the use of electronic medical records

hepatitis–inflammation of the liver

hyperglycemic hyperosmolar nonketotic syndrome–a diabetic syndrome characterized by excessive urination and dehydration

hypoglycemia–a lower-than-normal blood sugar level

mechanical index–the calculation used to identify the likelihood that cavitation could occur

nosocomial infection–a hospital-acquired infection

radiation forces–forces exerted by a sound beam on an absorber or reflector that can alter structures

shock–the body's pathologic response to illness, trauma, or severe physiologic or emotional stress

streaming–when acoustic fields cause motion of fluids

tachycardia–a heart rate that exceeds the normal rate for the age of the patient

thermal index–the calculation used to predict the maximum temperature elevation in tissues as a result of the attenuation of sound

PATIENT CARE, SAFETY, AND COMMUNICATION

Patient Identification, Documentation, and Verification of Requested Examinations

The correct identification of patients who require sonographic procedures is a fundamental, and yet crucial part of patient care. Sonographers should not limit the identification of a patient to simply asking the patient his or her last name. Verifying the patient's wristband information for identifying markers, which includes the patient's name, medical record number, and date of birth, is an essential part of patient care. All of this information should match with the requesting physician's and examination information. In some facilities, wristbands may have explicit colors that identify the patient as an outpatient or inpatient. Additionally, wristbands can indicate special precautions that should be taken for the concern of the patient and health care workers.

In 2003, the **Health Insurance Portability and Accountability Act** (HIPAA) became effective in the United States. These HIPAA privacy rules influence many aspects of patient care and ensure that patient records are kept private by establishing certain standards or safeguards (Table 6-1). HIPAA also included a special provision to ensure that electronic transactions are safely performed.

Sonographers can play a key role in the protection of sensitive patient information. Computer monitors should be out of the viewing area of patients. Images should be viewed in a private locale, away from high-traffic areas. If viewing of images takes place outside of the health care facility, as in the case of publication and in the educational setting, patient identification and all distinctive markers should be omitted from the images. The discussion of sonographic studies and patient history should take place in a private area. Patient confidentiality must never be compromised.

Proper documentation, both on the images obtained and of the procedure performed, is also crucial in the sequence of proper patient care. According to the American Institute of Ultrasound in Medicine (AIUM), documentation of ultrasound images should include the patient's name and other identifying information, including facility information, date of the sonographic examination, and image orientation. The postexamination sonographic worksheet should include, but not be limited to, the patient's name, the date and type of examination, relevant clinical information and/or ICD 9 code, the name of patient's health care provider, and any other appropriate contact information.

TABLE 6 - 1 HIPAA goals.
HIPAA attempts to:
• Establish new standards for the release of health records
• Protect health records by establishing new standards for health care professionals to follow
• Apply strict penalties for those who violate patient confidentiality and patient rights
• Provide more patient education

Patient Interaction, Effective Communication, and Obtaining a Clinical History

The role of the sonographer in patient care is critical. The sonographer should understand the physics of sound and should be able to relate to their patients the basic information about the use of ultrasound in medicines. Therefore, sonographers should not only be capable of performing sonographic examination but also be proficient in effectively communicating with their patients. An awareness of cultural diversity is essential, and sonographers should provide reasonable accommodations for those who have varying cultural or religious backgrounds.

Communication is the transfer of information from one person to another. It can be described as verbal or nonverbal. Verbal communication deals with spoken words. Picking the correct words to communicate with the patient is imperative. For example, the use of technical jargon may confuse the patient and result in the establishment of communication barriers. The details of the sonographic examination should be in clear, concise language and should always allow the opportunity for the patient to ask questions.

If a patient does not speak English, or national language, the sonographer should obtain an interpreter. This practice will ensure that the patient is completely informed about the procedure prior to the procedure taking place. Especially in these situations, nonverbal communication can aid as an effective means of communication. Nonverbal communication includes signs, hand gestures, facial expressions, and other body motions. Nevertheless, they should never completely take the place of verbal communication. Unfortunately, the risk of litigation increases if a patient is not thoroughly informed of the procedure prior to its initiation.

Obtaining a thorough patient history is also a significant step toward proper patient care. Clinical history should be discussed with the patient before the sonographic examination begins. One goal of the sonographer should be to perform clinical correlation with the sonographic images acquired throughout the examination. There are several general questions that can be asked to start a conversation with the patient who presents with pain and for those without noticeable pain (Tables 6-2 and 6-3). These questions should be followed by more in-depth questions, that are not necessarily leading questions, but rather open-ended, so as to obtain further information. If performed rationally, and in sequence, a clinical inquiry can often lead to not previously revealed clinical concerns that the patient may have. Other sources of clinical history exist, including archived imaging and diagnostic studies, laboratory findings, and family history.

TABLE 6-2 Clinical history questions for the patient who is complaining of pain.

Universal Clinical History Question for the Symptomatic Patient
• Where is the problem or area of pain?
• When did the pain start?
• How severe is the pain?
• What makes the pain go away or get worse?
• What else happens when the pain begins?

TABLE 6-3 Clinical history questions for the patient who is not complaining of pain.
Universal Clinical History Questions for the Asymptomatic Patient
• Are you a diabetic? • Do you have high blood pressure? • Do you smoke? • Do you take any medications? • Have you had any surgeries (related to the examination area)?

Emergency Situations

When emergency situations arise, sonographers must be prepared. Certification by the American Heart Association in cardiopulmonary resuscitation (CPR) should be maintained. CPR is most often used to counteract the effects of suspected cardiac arrest, or heart attack. The classic presentation of cardiac arrest includes a loss of consciousness, loss of blood pressure, dilation of the pupils, and possibly seizures. There are specific actions that the sonographer should be prepared to make in the presence of cardiac arrest (Table 6-4). If available, an **automatic external defibrillator** may be used to assess the patient's heart rhythm and administer a therapeutic shock, if necessary, to return the heart to normal rhythm.

Sonographers should also be prepared to efficiently react to patients who may experience shock. **Shock** is the body's pathologic response to illness, trauma, or severe physiologic or emotional stress. There are several different classifications of shock (Table 6-5). The initial clinical manifestation of shock may not be obvious. However, as the body responds to the effects of shock, clinical observations can be made. The compensatory patient will experience cold and clammy skin, decreased urine output, increased respiration, reduced bowel sounds, and increased anxiety. If shock is allowed to progress, the patient's blood pressure will drop, their respirations will decrease, and they will experience **tachycardia**, chest pain, and possibly have a loss of mental alertness. In the irreparable stage of shock, vital organs, such as the kidneys and liver, shut down and death is nearly unavoidable. The sonographer should immediately call for emergency assistance when any form of shock is suspected. They should also be prepared to perform CPR and assist with crash cart procedures.

TABLE 6-4 Sonographer's response to cardiac arrest.
Sonographer's Response to Cardiac Arrest
1. In the presence of an unresponsive patient, shake the patient and ask, "Are you okay?" 2. If there is no response, call a "code." 3. If no one is near, shout for help. 4. Do not leave the patient. 5. Check the carotid pulse of an adult patient. 6. If there is no pulse, place the patient in the supine position and begin performing CPR.

T A B L E 6 - 5 The classifications and explanation of shock.

Classification of Shock	Explanation
Anaphylactic shock	A subcategory of distributive shock that results from an exaggerated allergic reaction, leading to vasodilation and pooling in the peripheral blood vessels. It can be caused by medications, iodinated contrast agents that are often used in x-ray procedures, and insect venoms.
Cardiogenic shock	Failure of the heart to pump the proper amount of blood to the vital organs. It can be caused by myocardial infarction, cardiac tamponade, dysrhythmias, or other cardiac pathology.
Distributive shock	When the blood vessels lack the ability to constrict and assist in the return of blood to the heart, therefore leading to a pooling of peripheral blood. There are three types of distributive shock: neurogenic, septic, and anaphylactic.
Hypovolemic shock	When the amount of intravascular fluid decreases by 15% to 25%. It can be caused by internal or external hemorrhage, loss of plasma from burns, or fluid loss from vomiting, diarrhea, or medications.
Neurogenic shock	A subcategory of distributive shock in which there is a loss of the sympathetic tone causing vasodilation of the peripheral blood vessels. It can be caused by spinal cord injuries, severe pain, neurogenic damage, medications, lack of glucose, and adverse effects of anesthesia.
Obstructive shock	Results from pathologic conditions that interfere with the normal pumping action of the heart. It can be caused by pulmonary embolism, pulmonary hypertension, arterial stenosis, and possibly tumors that obstruct normal blood flow to the heart.
Septic shock	A subcategory of distributive shock in which there is an immune response of the body that leads to capillary permeability and vasodilation. It can be caused by invasive organisms, such as bacteria.

Some sonographic procedures require the patient to fast as part of preparation for the examination. Diabetic patients can be distinctly affected when they have not had anything to eat for an extended period of time. The sonographer should be aware if the patient is a diabetic, as these emergency situations may be treated differently. Patients with **diabetes mellitus** may suffer from three complications that the sonographer may have to recognize: **hypoglycemia, diabetic ketoacidosis**, and **hyperglycemic hyperosmolar nonketotic syndrome** (Table 6-6). Complications of diabetes include

T A B L E 6 - 6 Diabetic emergencies.

Acute Complication of Diabetes Mellitus	Explanation
Hypoglycemia	Occurs when a patient has an excess amount of insulin or oral hypoglycemic medication in their system. This may be seen in the diabetic patient who has had nothing to eat for several hours.
Diabetic ketoacidosis (hyperglycemia)	Occurs when a patient has insufficient insulin, resulting in excess glucose production by the liver.

tachycardia, headache, blurred vision, extreme thirst, polyuria, or a sweet odor to the breath (in diabetic ketoacidosis). The sonographer should immediately notify the radiologist, interpreting physician of the examination, or emergency room physician and be prepared to monitor the patient's vital signs or assist the emergency team in patient care procedures.

Infection Control and Universal Precautions

Health care workers can be exposed to various viruses during their daily practice. Hepatitis B and C viruses, human immunodeficiency virus (HIV), tuberculosis (TB), and methicillin-resistant Staphylococcus aureus (MRSA) are among the list of communicable diseases that may be transmitted in the hospital from a patient to a health care worker.

Toxins, certain drugs, some diseases, heavy alcohol use, and bacterial and viral infections can all cause **hepatitis**. Hepatitis B and C are transmitted via contact with infectious blood, semen, and other body fluids, from having sex with an infected person, sharing contaminated needles to inject drugs, or from an infected mother to her newborn. Hepatitis B vaccination is typically provided to all health care workers who may be exposed. It is a simple set of three injections. There is no present vaccine for hepatitis C.

HIV is the virus that leads to acquired immune deficiency syndrome (AIDS). It is spread by sexual contact with an infected person, by sharing needles with someone who is infected, through transfusions of infected blood or blood clotting factors, or through childbirth or breast milk. In the health care setting, workers have been infected with HIV after being stuck with needles containing HIV-infected blood, although the risk is minimal.

TB is an airborne disease found in the lungs, and possibly other organs, of an infected person. The TB bacteria are released from an infected individual most often when that person coughs, sneezes, speaks, or sings. People nearby, such as sonographers and other patients, may breathe in these bacteria and become infected. The TB skin test, the Mantoux tuberculin skin test, is performed to detect whether the individual is infected with TB. This test has been a mainstay in the detection and prevention of spread of TB in the health care setting.

MRSA is a type of staphylococcus or "staph" bacteria that is resistant to many antibiotics. MRSA has become a rampant malady spread through close personal contact in the health care setting. Unfortunately, it is the health care worker who may be the means of transmission of this destructive organism. Most staff infections manifest as an infected area on the skin.

Infection control, and consequently the reduction in the spread of infection, should be a priority in all sonography departments. The chain of infection begins with a pathogenic organism (Table 6-7) (Figure 6-1). Pathogens include viruses, fungi, and parasites. Pathogens need a reservoir to stay alive. The reservoir provides an environment in which the pathogen can grow or multiply. A reservoir could be found anywhere in the clinical setting, including on our hands, the ultrasound machine, and the examination table. Pathogens are also found in body fluids such as blood and urine, in the nose, and in the mouth. A portal of exit from the reservoir must be available for the pathogen to be transmitted to another individual. The mode of transmission by the hands is a common occurrence in the clinical environment.

TABLE **6-7** Chain of infection.

Chain of Infection
1. Infectious agent
2. Reservoir
3. Portal of exit
4. Mode of transmission
5. Portal of entry
6. Susceptible host

Although the use of gloves should be a routine part of patient care, the single most vital daily task that a sonographer can perform to prevent the spread of infection is the practice of regular hand washing. Hand washing, when performed accurately, can reduce the spread of infection between patients significantly. Although alcohol-based hand rubs may be easily accessible, they should never take the place of hand washing entirely. Hand washing should take place before and after any contact with patients.

The use of other personal protective equipment (PPE) such as gowns and masks is also an effective means of reducing the spread of infection. PPEs are considered to be transmission barriers. They help prevent the transportation of pathogens from the infected person to the general environment (Figure 6-2). There are also barrier techniques that can be used to prevent the spread of infection. These methods include sterilization, decontamination, and disposing of infected waste.

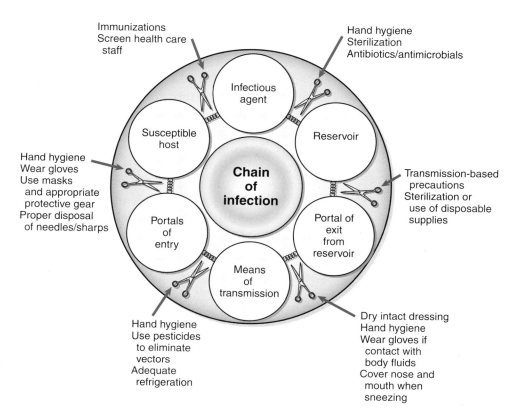

FIGURE 6-1 The infection cycle is demonstrated as a chain. The goal is to break the links of the chain to end the cycle. (Image adapted from Murphy D. Infectious microbes and disease: General principles. Nursing Spectrum. 1998;7(2):12–14.)

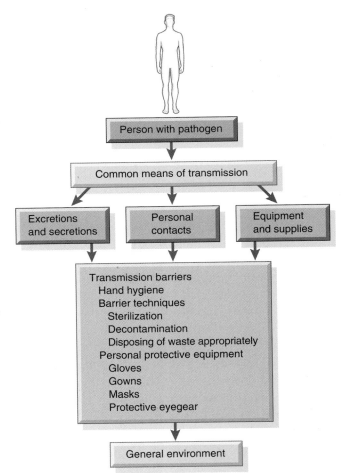

FIGURE 6-2 Transmission barriers help prevent the transporting of pathogens from the infected person to the general environment. Transmission barriers include hand hygiene, barrier techniques, and personal protective equipment. (Image reprinted with permission from Taylor CR, Carol Lillis RN, et al. Fundamentals of Nursing: The Art And Science Of Nursing Care. 6th Ed. Philadelphia: Lippincott Williams & Wilkins, 2008.)

The Occupational Safety and Health Administration and the Centers for Disease Control have established Standard Precaution, which may also be referred to as "Universal Precautions." These precautions deal with safety measures that should apply to blood, all body fluids, secretions, excretions, nonintact skin, and mucous membranes. They not only encourage safe practices when dealing with patients but also promote cleanliness in the health care setting.

A **nosocomial infection** is a hospital-acquired infection. One of the most widespread nosocomial infections is a urinary tract infection, caused by the incorrect use and placement of a Foley catheter bag. The bag, when placed above or at the level of the urinary bladder, could allow retrograde flow into the bladder from the catheter bag. To minimize the potential for a urinary tract infection, the patient's catheter bag should be placed below the level of the urinary bladder. As mentioned earlier, the spread of MRSA is also a rapidly growing problem in hospitals.

Disinfection of ultrasound equipment should be performed. Various materials may be used to clean the ultrasound equipment daily between patients. The transducer, the transducer cord, and the keyboard should all be cleaned with a disinfectant chemical. Endocavity transducers, such as transvaginal, transrectal, and transesophageal probes, are typically soaked in a glutaraldehyde-based solution or some form of cold-sterilizing solution for the manufacturers' suggested submersion time. The disinfectant of endocavity transducers should be well documented. These chemicals can be exceedingly hazardous to manage. Therefore, the PPE, as well as proper disposal techniques, must be employed.

BIOEFFECTS

According to the AIUM's *Prudent Use and Clinical Safety* statement, "No independently confirmed adverse effects caused by exposure from present diagnostic ultrasound instruments have been reported in human patients in the absence of contrast agents. Biologic effects (such as localized pulmonary bleeding) have been reported in mammalian systems at diagnostically relevant exposures but the clinical significance of such effects is not yet known. Ultrasound should be used by qualified health professionals to provide medical benefit to the patient."

ALARA

The AIUM formed and suggests the use of the ALARA principle: As Low As Reasonably Achievable. This term relates the amount of exposure time for the sonographer and patient during a diagnostic ultrasound examination. Although there are no proven biologic effects of diagnostic ranges of ultrasound on human tissue, this maxim encourages only the sensible use of ultrasound for diagnostic purposes. It is an acknowledgment and reminder that potential risks do exist and therefore exposure to high-frequency ultrasound should be curtailed. The official statement reads as follows:

> The potential benefits and risks of each examination should be considered. The ALARA (As Low As Reasonably Achievable) principle should be observed when adjusting controls that affect the acoustical output and by considering transducer dwell times.

Sound waves are attenuated in body tissues. Nonetheless, we know that sound can have both thermal (thermal mechanism) and nonthermal (nonthermal mechanism) effects on human tissues at certain intensities.

Thermal Mechanism and Thermal Index

As sound travels through the body, it is attenuated. The primary reason why tissue heats as sound is attenuated in the human body is absorption. Sound energy is converted to heat typically as a result of an increase in intensity and frequency. Elevation in the temperature of certain tissues can cause significant damage. For example, embryonic tissue constructing the heart may be extremely sensitive to subtle temperature changes. This elevation in local tissue temperature can be evaluated. The **thermal index** is a calculation used to predict the maximum temperature elevation in tissues as a result of the attenuation of sound. The maximum heating of tissue is related to the sound beams spatial pulse temporal average (SPTA). The official AIUM statement reads: "No effects have been observed for an unfocused beam having free-field SPTA intensities below 100 mW/cm^2, or a focused beam having intensities below 1 W/cm^2, or thermal index values of less than 2." It is important to remember that absorption is greater in bone than in soft tissue.

FIGURE 6-3 Cavitation. As ultrasound travels through tissues (top), it causes alternating compression and rarefaction, respectively (middle). Gas is drawn out of a solution during rarefaction, creating bubbles. These bubbles can fluctuate in size in a stable fashion with the changing tissue pressure. However, they may collapse. This collapse can result in local energy release and a focal increase in temperature at the microscopic level (bottom).

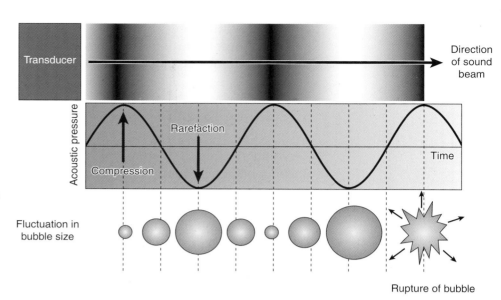

Nonthermal Mechanism and Mechanical Index

Nonthermal mechanisms include **radiation forces**, **streaming**, and **acoustic cavitation**, with the latter being the most worrisome. Nonthermal mechanisms may also be referred to as mechanical mechanisms. Cavitation is the action of an acoustic field within a fluid to generate bubbles (Figure 6-3). There are two types of cavitation: stable and transient. Stable cavitation produces bubbles that oscillate, or fluctuate, in size but do not rupture. Transient cavitation, also referred to as collapse, has the potential of causing the most biologic damage. With transient cavitation, larger bubbles are produced and subsequently rupture. The rupture of these bubbles produces a shock wave and an increase in tissue temperature in that area. This increase in temperature has been associated with biologic effects.

The **mechanical index** was developed to assist in evaluating the likelihood of cavitation to occur. However, the AIUM states, "In tissues that contain well-defined gas bodies, e.g., lung, no effects have been observed for in situ peak rarefactional pressures below approximately 0.4 MPa or mechanical index values less than approximately 0.4." Therefore, diagnostic ultrasound is not associated with an increase in biologic tissue damage.

REVIEW QUESTIONS

1. What term and philosophy relates the amount of exposure time for the sonographer and patient during a diagnostic ultrasound examination?
   a. Nonthermal mechanisms
   b. Mechanical mechanism
   c. As Low As Reasonably Achievable
   d. Health Insurance Portability and Accountability Act

2. Sonographers should verify the patient's wristband information for identifying markers. This includes which of the following?
   a. Patient's race
   b. Medical record number

    c. Date of registration
    d. Birth place

3. If a patient does not speak English, or the national language, the sonographer should:
    a. Use picture cards
    b. Cancel the examination
    c. Provide an interpreter
    d. Offer the patient paper and use hand gestures

4. The diabetic syndrome characterized by excessive urination and dehydration is:
    a. Hyperglycemic hyperosmolar nonketotic syndrome
    b. Hypoglycemic ketotic syndrome
    c. Ketoacidosis syndrome
    d. Diabetic ketoacidosis syndrome

5. What term is defined as the body's pathologic response to illness, trauma, or severe physiologic or emotional stress?
    a. Virus
    b. Shock
    c. Cardiac arrest
    d. Stroke

6. Which of the following would not be considered a part of the classic presentation of cardiac arrest?
    a. Headache
    b. Loss of consciousness
    c. Loss of blood pressure
    d. Dilation of the pupils

7. Which of the following would be considered the best way to prevent the spread of infection?
    a. Covering your mouth when you cough
    b. Cleaning the ultrasound machine
    c. Hand washing
    d. Taking vitamins

8. What is defined as the action of an acoustic field within a fluid to generate bubbles?
    a. Thermal index
    b. Cavitation
    c. Dehydration
    d. Streaming

9. What is it called when an acoustic field causes motion of fluids?
    a. Streaming
    b. Cavitation
    c. Hydrostatic pressure
    d. Radiation forces

10. The calculation used to predict the maximum temperature elevation in tissues as a result of attenuation of sound is the:
    a. Spatial temporal index
    b. Nonmechanical index
    c. Mechanical index
    d. Thermal index

11. The maximum heating of tissue is related to the sound beams:
    a. Spatial average peak average
    b. Spatial pulse temporal average
    c. Spatial average temporal average
    d. Spatial average

12. The Health Insurance Portability and Accountability Act attempts to do all of the following except:
    a. Establish new standards for the release of health records.
    b. Protect health records by establishing new standards for health care professionals to follow.
    c. Apply strict penalties for those who violate patient confidentiality and patient rights.
    d. Encourage safe practices when dealing with patients; they also promote cleanliness in the health care setting.

13. Which of the following is defined as forces exerted by a sound beam on an absorber or reflector that can alter structures?
    a. Cavitation
    b. Radioactive mechanism
    c. Radiation forces
    d. Nonmechanical strengths

14. Which of the following forms of cavitation has the most potential for inducing biologic damage?
    a. Acute
    b. Chronic
    c. Transient
    d. Stable

15. The calculation used to assist in evaluating the likelihood of cavitation to occur is referred to as the:
    a. Cavitational index
    b. Mechanical index
    c. Nonmechanical index
    d. Thermal index

16. Which of the following would be best described as the failure of the heart to pump the proper amount of blood to the vital organs?
    a. Distributive shock
    b. Neurogenic shock
    c. Hypovolemic shock
    d. Cardiogenic shock

17. A nosocomial infection is best described as a:
    a. Hospital-acquired infection
    b. Infection caused by not washing your hands
    c. A nasal infection spread by sneezing
    d. An airborne disease found in infected persons' lungs that is spread by coughing

18. Which of the following could be a cause of anaphylactic shock?
    a. Cardiac tamponade
    b. Diarrhea
    c. Iodinated contrast agents
    d. Lack of glucose

19. Which of the following would be considered one of the most common nosocomial infections?
    a. AIDS
    b. Hepatitis B
    c. Urinary tract infections
    d. Tuberculosis

20. An infectious agent needs to initially have which of the following to grow and survive?
    a. Means of transmission
    b. Portal of entry
    c. Portal of exit
    d. Reservoir

21. Which of the following would not be considered a common virus that a health care worker would be exposed to?
    a. Hepatitis B
    b. Hepatitis C
    c. Methicillin-resistant Staphylococcus aureus
    d. Hepatitis K

22. Which of the following would not be considered a transmission barrier that would help prevent the transporting of pathogens from the infected person to the general environment?
    a. Gloves
    b. Hand washing
    c. Needles
    d. Sterilization

23. Universal or standard precautions apply to all of the following except:
    a. Sweat
    b. Nonintact skin
    c. Blood
    d. Pleural fluid

24. When viewing sonographic images outside of the clinical arena, all of the following information are required to be removed except:
    a. Patient's name
    b. Facility
    c. Date
    d. Image orientation

25. Which of the following is best described as an airborne disease that is spread by bacteria released from an infected individual when that person coughs, sneezes, speaks, or sings?
    a. Methicillin-resistant Staphylococcus aureus
    b. Hepatitis B
    c. Tuberculosis
    d. Hepatitis C

26. Which of the following would most likely manifest as a weeping skin lesion that is swollen and infected?
    a. Methicillin-resistant Staphylococcus aureus
    b. Tuberculosis
    c. Human immunodeficiency virus
    d. Hepatitis C

27. Hepatitis denotes:
    a. Liver inflammation
    b. Renal disorders
    c. Metabolic obstruction
    d. Biliary infection

28. All of the following are considered to be part of nonthermal mechanisms of biologic effects except:
    a. Radiation forces
    b. Streaming
    c. Acoustic cavitation
    d. Tissue heating

29. What is considered to be the primary reason why tissue heats as sound is attenuated in the human body?
    a. Reflection
    b. Enhancement
    c. Cavitation
    d. Absorption

30. No biologic effects have been observed for an unfocused beam having free-field SPTA intensities below:
    a. 100 mW/cm^2
    b. 10 W/cm^2
    c. 1000 mW/ cm^2
    d. 1540 m/s

31. Which of the following would be most likely caused by an arterial stenosis?
    a. Nosocomial infection
    b. Cardiogenic shock
    c. Hypovolemic shock
    d. Obstructive shock

32. Which of the following would be described as a complication of diabetes that results from a severe lack of insulin, in which case the patient's breath may have a sweet smell?
    a. Hyperglycemic hyperosmolar nonketotic syndrome
    b. Diabetic ketoacidosis
    c. Hypovolemic shock
    d. Hypoglycemia

33. In tissues that contain well-defined gas bodies, no effects have been observed for in situ peak rarefactional pressures below a mechanical index value less than approximately:
    a. 0.4
    b. 0.8
    c. 2
    d. 100

34. No effects have been observed for an unfocused beam having thermal index value of less than:
    a. 0.4
    b. 0.8
    c. 2
    d. 100

35. Which of the following is required in order for a pathogen to be transmitted from one individual to another?
    a. Gateway of admission
    b. Portal of exit
    c. Infectious agent
    d. Vulnerable agent

36. Which of the following is not transmitted via contact with infectious blood or accidental needle sticks?
    a. Tuberculosis
    b. Human immunodeficiency virus
    c. Hepatitis C
    d. Hepatitis B

37. Which of the following would not be considered a clinical complication of diabetes mellitus?
    a. Blurred vision
    b. Extreme thirst
    c. Sweet odor to the breath
    d. Decreased urine output

38. Human immunodeficiency virus is spread by all of the following means except:
    a. Sexual contact
    b. Kissing
    c. Needle stick
    d. Blood transfusion

39. Some clinical manifestation of shock includes all of the following except:
    a. Clammy skin
    b. Decreased urine output
    c. Increased anxiety
    d. Extreme thirst

40. Which of the following statements is not true concerning hand washing?
    a. Alcohol-based hand rubs should be used to take the place of hand washing.
    b. Hand washing should occur before and after any contact with patients.
    c. Hand washing is an effective means to prevent the spread of infection.
    d. Alcohol-based hand rubs should be used in conjunction with hand washing.

41. In the presence of a nonresponsive adult patient, which pulse should be evaluated?
    a. Radial
    b. Tibial
    c. Carotid
    d. Temporal

42. Personal protective equipment includes all of the following except:
    a. Gloves
    b. Gluteraldehyde soaking solution
    c. Gowns
    d. Face masks

43. Which of the following would not be considered a barrier technique?
    a. Sterilization
    b. Decontamination

c. Disposing of waste material

d. Hand hygiene

44. What would be the most likely means of transmission of the human immunodeficiency virus from a patient to a sonographer?

a. Exposure to fecal material

b. Holding the patient's hand without a glove

c. Needle stick

d. Coughing

45. What would be the most likely means of transmission of tuberculosis from a patient to a sonographer?

a. Exposure to fecal material

b. Holding the patient's hand without a glove

c. Needle stick

d. Coughing

46. Nonthermal mechanisms may also be referred to as:

a. Thermal mechanisms

b. Mechanical mechanisms

c. Thermal indices

d. Absorption influence

47. Which of the following would not be a subcategory of distributive shock?

a. Septic shock

b. Anaphylactic shock

c. Nosocomial shock

d. Neurogenic shock

48. Which of the following statements is true concerning the biologic effects of diagnostic ultrasound?

a. No effects caused by exposure from present diagnostic ultrasound instruments have been reported in human patients in the absence of contrast agents.

b. Very few biologic effects caused by exposure from diagnostic ultrasound instruments have been reported.

c. Biologic effects have been recognized and the risk and benefits must be considered for each examination.

d. The only biologic effect of diagnostic ultrasound exposure is cavitation.

49. All of the following are true statements about the use of gloves except:

a. Gloves should be used when there is any expected contact with infected materials.

b. Gloves can be used to replace hand washing.

c. Gloves should be changed between patients.

d. Gloves are considered personal protective equipment.

50. Which of the following best describes transient cavitation?

a. The type of cavitation in which there is a production of cavernous spaces within tissue.

b. The type of cavitation that produces bubbles that oscillate, or fluctuate, in size but do not rupture.

c. The type of cavitation in which bubbles do not exist.

d. The type of cavitation when larger bubbles are produced and subsequently rupture.

SUGGESTED READINGS

American Institute of Ultrasound in Medicine Web site. Available at: http://www.aium.org/publications/statements.aspx; http://www.aium.org/publications/guidelines/documentation.pdf.

Center for Disease Control. Available at: http://www.cdc.gov/.

Craig M. Essentials of Sonography and Patient Care. 2nd Ed. St. Louis, MO: Saunders, 2006.

Edelman SK. Understanding Ultrasound Physics. 3rd Ed. Woodlands, TX: ESP Inc., 2005.

Kremkau FW. Diagnostic Ultrasound: Principles and Instruments. 7th Ed. St. Louis, MO: Saunders, 2006.

Rumack C, Wilson S, Charboneau J. Diagnostic Ultrasound. St. Louis, MO: Mosby, 2005.

Torres L, Dutton A, Linn-Watson T. Patient Care in Imaging Technology. 7th Ed. Baltimore, MD: Lippincott Williams and Wilkins, 2010.

Registry Review Exam

This section provides a complete registry review examination, with answers and rationales at the end. In addition, a registry review exam simulator is provided online. Using the access ID provided on the inside front cover of this book to access thePoint at **thepoint.lww.com/product/isbn/9781608311378**, the reader can take computer-based examinations with more intense "registry-like" questions. With more than 300 additional questions, the exam simulator provides a new mock exam every time the user logs in.

1. What type of wave is sound?
   a. Mechanical, transverse
   b. Mechanical, longitudinal
   c. Transverse, longitudinal
   d. Lateral wave

2. The frequency ranges for ultrasound are:
   a. <20 Hz
   b. 20 to 20,000 Hz
   c. >20 kHz
   d. >2000 HZ

3. The speed of sound in soft tissue is:
   a. 1.54 mm/s
   b. 1540 m/s
   c. 1540 km/s
   d. 1.54 m/μs

4. Which of the following transducers fires the elements in groups?
   a. Linear sequenced array
   b. Phased array
   c. Mechanical sector
   d. Linear phased array

5. The unit for wavelength is:
   a. Millimeters
   b. Hertz
   c. Microseconds
   d. Milliliters

6. Enhancement is caused by:
   a. Strongly reflecting structures
   b. Propagation speed errors
   c. Snell's law
   d. Weakly attenuating structures

7. The wavelength in a material having a propagation speed of 1.5 mm/μs employing a transducer frequency of 5.0 MHZ is:
   a. 0.3 mm
   b. 0.3 cm
   c. 0.6 mm
   d. 3.0 mm

8. An ultrasound transducer converts:
   a. Electrical energy into light and heat
   b. Electrical energy into mechanical energy
   c. Mechanical energy into radiation
   d. Sound into ultrasound

9. Arrange the following media in correct order from the lowest attenuation to highest.
   a. Air, fat, muscle, bone
   b. Muscle, fat, air, bone
   c. Fat, muscle, bone, air
   d. Muscle, air, fat, bone

10. Arrange the following media in terms of propagation speed, from lowest to highest.
    a. Air, fat, muscle, bone
    b. Bone, fat, air, muscle
    c. Bone, muscle, fat, air
    d. Muscle, air, fat, bone

11. If the frequency doubles, what happens to the wavelength?
    a. Increases fourfold
    b. Increases twofold
    c. Decreases by one half
    d. Frequency has no relationship to wavelength

12. What happens to intensity if the amplitude of a signal is halved?
    a. Quartered
    b. Quadrupled
    c. Halved
    d. No change

13. Which of the following would be used to describe the percentage of time that sound is on?
    a. Intensity
    b. Amplitude
    c. SPTA
    d. Duty factor

14. A 3 dB gain would indicate an increase in intensity by:
    a. 2 times
    b. 4 times
    c. 8 times
    d. 10 times

15. Ignoring the effects of attenuation, the intensity of the ultrasound beam is usually greater at the focal zone because of:
    a. Decreased attenuation
    b. The smaller beam diameter
    c. Diffraction effects
    d. A shorter duty factor

16. Attenuation denotes:
    a. Progressive weakening of the sound beam as it travels
    b. Density of tissue and the speed of sound in the tissues
    c. The redirection of the ultrasound back to the transducer
    d. Bending of the transmitted wave after crossing an interface

17. Which of the following has the lowest intensity?
    a. SPTP
    b. SATP
    c. SPTA
    d. SATA

18. What is the definition of the beam uniformity ratio?
    a. The spatial intensity divided by the spatial peak intensity
    b. The spatial peak intensity divided by the spatial average intensity
    c. The temporal average intensity divided by the spatial average intensity
    d. The temporal peak intensity divided by the spatial peak intensity

19. Continuous-wave Doppler has a duty factor of:
    a. <1%
    b. 100%
    c. >100%
    d. 50%

20. The spatial pulse length is defined as the product of the _____ and the number of _____ in a pulse?
    a. Cycles, frequency
    b. Frequency, velocity
    c. Wavelength, cycles
    d. Frequency, wavelength

21. With phased array transducers, the transmitted sound beam is steered by:
    a. Mechanically sweeping the piezoelectric elements
    b. Mechanically rotating the piezoelectric elements
    c. Varying the timing of pulses to the individual piezoelectric elements
    d. Varying the frequency of pulses to the individual piezoelectric elements

22. If the gain of an amplifier is 18 dB, what is the new gain if the power is reduced by half?
    a. 15 dB
    b. 9 dB
    c. 36 dB
    d. 0.5 dB

23. Which of the following is true?
    a. SPTA is always equal to or greater than SPTP
    b. SPTP is always equal to or greater than SPTA
    c. SATA is always equal to or greater than SATP
    d. SPTA is equal to or greater than SPTP

24. If the amplitude of a wave is increased threefold, the power will:
    a. Decrease threefold
    b. Increase threefold
    c. Increase ninefold
    d. Increase sixfold

25. Ultrasound attenuates an average of _____dB/cm of travel for each megahertz of frequency.
    a. 1
    b. 0.7
    c. 0.33
    d. 0.25

26. If the intensity transmission coefficient is 0.74, the intensity reflection coefficient will be:
    a. 1.06
    b. 6.00
    c. 0.26
    d. 0.04

27. Acoustic impedance is defined as the product of:
    a. The mismatch between two interfaces
    b. A change in velocity at oblique incidence
    c. The speed of sound in tissue and density of the tissue
    d. The wavelength and frequency

28. Rayleigh scattering is an example of:
    a. A reflector whose size is smaller than the wavelength
    b. A reflector whose size is significantly larger than the wavelength
    c. A specular reflection
    c. A type of side lobe artifact

29. If medium 2 impedance is equal to medium 1 impedance:
    a. 100% of the intensity will be reflected
    b. 100% of the intensity will be transmitted
    c. The reflection and transmission coefficients will be equal
    d. The answer cannot be determined without values given

30. What is the total attenuation of a 3.5-MHz pulse after passing through 2 cm of soft tissue?
    a. 7 dB
    b. 3.5 dB
    c. 17 dB
    d. 1.75 dB

31. The thinner the piezoelectric element,
    a. The lower the frequency
    b. The higher the frequency
    c. The higher the amplitude
    d. The lower the amplitude

32. The unit for impedance is:
    a. dB
    b. mW/cm^2
    c. Rayls
    d. No units

33. A sound beam encounters an interface at a 90° angle. If the speed of sound in the first tissue is 1540 m/s and the speed of sound in the second tissue is 1450 m/s, which of the following numbers most closely approximates the angle of beam transmission?
    a. <90°
    b. 90°

c. >90°
d. Need the impedance to compute angle of transmission

34. ALARA stands for:
a. As low as reasonably achievable
b. As long as reasonably acceptable
c. As little as reasonably allowable
d. As long as reasonably achievable

35. A decibel (dB) describes the:
a. Ratio of two sound intensities
b. Sum of two sound intensities
c. Amount of scattering
d. Velocity of the sound wave

36. The correct equation for Snell's law is:
a. $R = (Z_2 - Z_1)^2/(Z_2 + Z_1)^2$
b. $Z = pc$
c. $\sin \theta_t = (C_2/C_1) \times \sin \theta_i$
d. $Fd = 2fv\cos \theta/c$

37. The attenuation coefficient of sound in soft tissue can be defined by which of the following equations?
a. One half the frequency times the path length
b. Frequency/6
c. Frequency/2
d. Frequency × 2

38. The intensity transmission coefficient is equal to:
a. 1 + intensity reflection coefficient
b. 1 − intensity reflection coefficient
c. The square of the angle of transmission
d. (Intensity transmission coefficient)/2

39. The range equation explains:
a. Side lobes
b. Distance to reflector
c. Attenuation
d. Calibration

40. The typical value for attenuation coefficient for 6 MHz ultrasound in soft tissue is:
a. 3 dB/cm
b. 1 dB/cm/Hz
c. 3 dB/cm²
d. 2 dB

41. What must be known in order to calculate distance to a reflector?
a. Attenuation, propagation speed, density
b. Attenuation, impedance
c. Travel time, propagation speed
d. Density, propagation speed

42. Specular reflections:
a. Occur when the interface is larger than the wavelength
b. Occur when the interface is smaller than the wavelength
c. Arise from interfaces smaller than 3 mm
d. Are not dependent on the angle of incidence

43. What is the reflected intensity from a boundary between two materials if the incident intensity is 1 mW/cm² and the impedances are 25 and 75?
    a. 0.25 mW/cm²
    b. 0.33 mW/cm²
    c. 0.50 mW/cm²
    d. 1.0 mW/cm²

44. The layer of material within the transducer which has an intermediate impedance between the transducer element and human tissue is known as the:
    a. Filler medium
    b. Damping medium
    c. Acoustic medium
    d. Matching layer

45. Which of the following relates bandwidth to operating frequency?
    a. Near zone
    b. Piezoelectric crystal
    c. Quality factor
    d. Far zone

46. The piezoelectric effect can best be described as:
    a. Density of tissue and the speed of sound in the tissues
    b. Mechanical deformation that results from a high voltage applied to the face of the crystal that in turn generates a pressure wave
    c. Having a damaging effect on crystal due to high voltage
    d. The decrease in intensity that results from the application of a damping material

47. Which of the following are most commonly used in ultrasound transducers?
    a. Lead zirconate titanate
    b. Barium sulfate
    c. Epoxy loaded with tungsten
    d. Quartz

48. Diffraction refers to:
    a. Spreading out of the ultrasound beam
    b. Conversion of sound to heat
    c. Redirection of a portion of the sound from a boundary beam
    d. Bending of the sound beam crossing a boundary

49. The method for sterilizing transducers is:
    a. Heat sterilization
    b. Steam
    c. Cold sterilization
    d. Autoclave

50. A transducer with which frequency would have the thickest element(s)?
    a. 2 MHz
    b. 3.5 MHz
    c. 5 MHz
    d. 7.5 MHz

51. Which of the following is best defined as the ability to discriminate between two closely spaced reflectors?
    a. Definition
    b. Range accuracy
    c. Spatial resolution
    d. Amplification

52. Which of the following is an effect of focusing?
    a. Improved lateral resolution
    b. Improved axial resolution
    c. Increased beam divergence
    d. Higher frequency

53. Bandwidth is:
    a. A source of artifacts
    b. A potential shade of gray
    c. The range of frequencies produced by the transducer
    d. Undesirable interference or noise

54. Within the same medium using the same transducer, decreasing the _____ decreases the beam diameter in the _____.
    a. Frequency, far zone
    b. Wavelength, far zone
    c. Frequency, near zone
    d. Intensity, far zone

55. The acoustic impedance of the transducer's matching layer:
    a. Is chosen to improve transmission into the body
    b. Is chosen to have increased internal reflections
    c. Determines the frequency
    d. None of the above

56. If the amount of damping decreases, the bandwidth:
    a. Stays the same
    b. Increases
    c. Decreases
    d. Damping and bandwidth are unrelated

57. The region where the sound beam is the smallest is referred to as the:
    a. Fresnel spot
    b. Focus
    c. Near field
    d. Far field

58. The near zone length is determined by:
    a. Number of focal zones
    b. Frame rate
    c. Pulse repetition frequency
    d. Transducer frequency

59. The type of transducer that utilizes concentric rings is called:
    a. Sequential array
    b. Phased array
    c. Annular array
    d. Spatial array

60. A wave's initial intensity is 2 mW/cm^2. There is an increase of 10 dB. What is the final intensity?
    a. 4 mW/cm^3
    b. 8 mW/cm^2
    c. 12 mW/cm^2
    d. 20 mW/cm^2

61. Which of the following is described best as a transducer that has multiple elements in a curved shape?
    a. Annular array
    b. Mechanical sector
    c. Curvilinear
    d. Linear array

62. What is the name of the control that compensates for attenuation related to path length?
    a. Near gain
    b. Far gain
    c. TGC
    d. Reject

63. The echoes are stored before final display by the:
    a. Receiver
    b. Scan converter
    c. Demodulator
    d. Transducer

64. What portion of the ultrasound system drives the transducer?
    a. Pulser
    b. Receiver
    c. Scan converter
    d. TGC controls

65. What component of the ultrasound system contains the digital-to-analog converter?
    a. Scan converter
    b. Pulser
    c. Receiver
    d. Display

66. How many different shades of gray can the human eye discern at one time?
    a. 16
    b. 32
    c. 64
    d. 100

67. Most current ultrasound systems have _____ shades of gray available.
    a. 4
    b. 32
    c. 64
    d. 256

68. How many bits per pixel can be displayed with 4 bits of memory?
    a. 2
    b. 4
    c. 8
    d. 16

69. The spatial resolution capabilities of the system are mainly functions of the:
    a. Pulser
    b. Transducer
    c. Receiver
    d. Display

70. The echo intensity on a grayscale of 32 shades is represented by the binary number:
    a. 10101
    b. 1010
    c. 100000
    d. 110000

71. Preprocessing of the information that is fed to the scan converter:
    a. Enlarges each pixel to provide a magnified image
    b. Determines the CRT brightness assigned to stored grayscale levels
    c. Determines the assignment of echoes to predetermined gray levels
    d. Determines the grayscale emphasis of stored gray levels

72. Which of the following do grayscale systems typically use as a means of signal dynamic range reduction?
    a. Rejection
    b. Compression
    c. Relaxation
    d. Elimination

73. Area is expressed by which of the following units?
    a. m/s
    b. cm
    c. cm^2
    d. cm^3

74. If the frequency of a transducer is increased, which of the following will decrease?
    a. Wavelength
    b. Propagation speed
    c. Pulse repetition frequency
    d. Pulse repetition period

75. With tissue harmonic imaging,
    a. The propagating pressure wave causes the sound to appear as a sinusoidal waveform
    b. The propagating pressure wave causes the sound to appear as a synovial waveform
    c. There are increased artifacts in the near field
    d. There are decreased artifacts in the near field

76. Which of the following is in the range of infrasound?
    a. 1.5 kHZ
    b. 15 Hz
    c. 25 Hz
    d. 1 MHz

77. Which of the following is in the range of audible sound?
    a. 15 Hz
    b. 18 kHz
    c. 25,000 Hz
    d. 2 Hz

78. Which of the following can be changed by the operator?
a. Frequency
b. Wavelength
c. Propagation speed
d. Pulse repetition frequency

79. Which of the following is the time it takes for one cycle to occur?
a. Period
b. Frequency
c. Wavelength
d. Pulse repetition period

80. The length of the pulse is the:
a. Period
b. Wavelength
c. Pulse repetition frequency
d. Spatial pulse length

81. Assuming oblique angle of incidence, if the propagation speed of medium 1 is greater than the propagation speed of medium 2, what will the angle of transmission be?
a. Greater than the angle of incidence
b. Less than the angle of incidence
c. Equal to the angle of incidence
d. Propagation speed does not influence the angle of transmission

82. A 5-MHz wave travels through 5 cm of soft tissue. If a 3.5-MHz transducer is selected instead, what happens to the propagation speed of the medium?
a. Increases
b. Decreases
c. No change
d. Not enough information given

83. The slowest propagation speed is found in which medium?
a. Bone
b. Air
c. Muscle
d. Liver

84. Which of the following represents the strength of the beam?
a. Frequency
b. Intensity
c. Q-factor
d. Duty factor

85. Which of the following is the unit of pressure amplitude?
a. W/cm^2
b. mm
c. mW
d. Pascal

86. Which of the following is the unit of intensity?
a. W/cm^2
b. mW
c. Pascal
d. W/cm

87. What else changes with a change in amplitude?
    a. Resonating frequency
    b. Output power
    c. Wavelength
    d. Spatial pulse length

88. Which of the following will increase the acoustic exposure to the patient?
    a. Increased receiver amplification
    b. Increased time gain compensation
    c. Decreased pulse repetition frequency
    d. Increased output gain

89. Which operator control adjusts the intensity of the transmitted pulse?
    a. Receiver gain
    b. Depth of scanning
    c. Power (dB)
    d. Time gain compensation (TGC)

90. What happens to the power if the intensity is doubled?
    a. No change
    b. It doubles
    c. It quadruples
    d. It is halved

91. The number of pulses that occur in 1 second is the:
    a. Pulse repetition frequency
    b. Pulse repetition period
    c. Pulse duration
    d. Duty factor

92. What is along the x-axis on a spectral Doppler waveform?
    a. Depth
    b. Amplitude
    c. Time
    d. Velocity

93. What is the unit of spatial pulse length?
    a. μs
    b. m
    c. m/s
    d. m/s^2

94. What testing device is used to measure acoustic output (intensity) level?
    a. Tissue phantom
    b. AIUM test phantom
    c. Doppler flow phantom
    d. Hydrophone

95. What is the principle that states sound waves are the result of the interference of many wavelets produced at the face of the transducer?
    a. Doppler's principle
    b. Bernoulli's principle
    c. Huygen's principle
    d. Poiseuille's principle

96. In what mode is the amplitude of the return echo represented by spikes along the *y*-axis of the image?
    a. M-mode
    b. C-mode
    c. B-mode
    d. A-mode

97. In B-mode imaging, amplitude is located on the __ -axis of the image
    a. *x*
    b. *y*
    c. *z*
    d. *c*

98. Which of the following determines the radial resolution of a system?
    a. PRF
    b. Impedance
    c. SPL
    d. Duty factor

99. The axial resolution can be improved by decreasing the _____ or increasing the _____.
    a. Impedance, pulse duration
    b. Number of cycles in a pulse, wavelength
    c. Propagation speed, spatial pulse length
    d. Number of cycles in a pulse, frequency

100. Two reflectors are 1.3 mm apart in a plane that is parallel to the beam. The SPL of the transducer is 2.6 mm. These two reflectors:
    a. Will show up as one dot on the screen
    b. Will show up as two dots on the screen
    c. Will not show up on the image at all
    d. Will have poor lateral resolution

101. In what zone does beam divergence occur?
    a. At the face of the transducer
    b. Focal zone
    c. Fraunhofer zone
    d. Fresnel zone

102. The larger the aperture,
    a. The shorter the near zone
    b. The longer the near zone
    c. The more divergence there is in far field
    d. The shorter the Fresnel zone

103. The ability to resolve two reflectors that lie parallel to the beam is the _____ resolution of a system
    a. Axial
    b. Lateral
    c. Elevational
    d. Temporal

104. The more focal zones used,
    a. The better the temporal resolution
    b. The worse the temporal resolution
    c. The better the axial resolution
    d. The better the SPL

105. In the most common type of transducers, the slice-thickness plane is focused:
    a. Using a lens
    b. Using a matrix array
    c. Electronically
    d. Using 2D technology

106. If sound travels through a large quantity of water and then encounters a reflector, the reflector will appear to be:
    a. Too far away
    b. Too close
    c. In the correct location
    d. Not enough information to tell

107. What is the maximum temperature increase below which there should be no thermally induced biologic effects?
    a. 95°C
    b. 10°C
    c. 4°C
    d. 2°C

108. Two sound beams with different frequencies are traveling through the same medium. Which beam will travel faster?
    a. The higher frequency sound
    b. The lower frequency sound
    c. Both will travel at the same speed
    d. Cannot be determined

109. A video display that is limited to only black and white, with no other shades of gray, is called:
    a. Binary
    b. Monochrome
    c. Bistable
    d. Unichrome

110. What is the name for the smallest amount of digital storage?
    a. The bit
    b. The pixel
    c. The byte
    d. The megabyte

111. In the Fresnel zone,
    a. The beam diameter is a constant
    b. The beam diameter diverges
    c. The beam area increases with distance from the transducer
    d. The beam area decreases with distance from the transducer

112. Information that travels to the scan converter from the receiver is initially in what format?
    a. Analog
    b. Digital
    c. Both
    d. Neither

113. Which of the following is true about color Doppler?
    a. Each pixel can be both color and grayscale at the same time
    b. Each pixel can either be grayscale or color
    c. Pixels cannot be colorized
    d. The gain determines the color priority of the pixels

114. Which of the following preserves the pixel density when enlarging the image?
    a. Read zoom
    b. Write magnification
    c. Max zoom
    d. Postprocessing magnification

115. What is the relationship between amplitude and frequency?
    a. Directly related
    b. Inversely related
    c. No relation
    d. Sometimes they are related, sometimes not

116. What is the relationship between spatial pulse length and pulse duration?
    a. Directly related
    b. Inversely related
    c. No relation
    d. Sometimes they are related, sometimes not

117. Which of the following is true about axial resolution?
    a. It decreases with depth
    b. It increases with depth
    c. It does not vary with depth
    d. It is best at the focal zone

118. If the _____ is increased, the flow increases.
    a. Pressure differential
    b. Resistance
    c. Length of vessel
    d. Viscosity of blood

119. Which law describes the relationship between flow and the pressure differential, viscosity, and length?
    a. Bernoulli's law
    b. Poiseuille's law
    c. Snell's law
    d. Doppler's law

120. The most common type of flow found in the body is:
    a. Plug
    b. Turbulent
    c. Laminar
    d. Chaotic

Answer Key for Registry Review Exam

1. b. Sound is a mechanical, longitudinal wave
2. c. Ultrasound is defined as sound with a frequency >20,000 Hz (20 kHz)
3. b. Sound travels through soft tissue at 1540 m/s
4. a. The linear sequenced array fires the elements in groups
5. a. Wavelength is a distance, therefore the unit must be a unit of distance such as millimeters
6. d. Enhancement occurs when sound passes through a weakly attenuating structure, such as a cyst
7. a. Wavelength = c/f. Therefore, 1.5 mm/μs ÷ 5 MHz = 0.3 mm
8. b. Ultrasound transducers convert mechanical energy into electrical energy and vice versa
9. c. The order of attenuation is: fat, muscle, bone, air. Air is the highest attenuator of ultrasound
10. a. Note that this order is for propagation speed, not attenuation. Air has the slowest propagation speed and bone has the highest
11. c. Frequency and wavelength are inversely related
12. a. Intensity is proportional to the amplitude squared, so if the amplitude is halved, the resulting intensity is one fourth the original intensity
13. d. Duty factor is the percentage of time the sound is being transmitted
14. a. A gain of 3 dB results in doubling of intensity (or power)
15. b. Intensity equals power divided by area. The area is smallest in the focal zone; therefore, the intensity is the highest (assuming no attenuation)
16. a. Attenuation is the weakening of the strength of the beam, typically from absorption, reflection, or scattering
17. d. SATA is the lowest of the intensities
18. b. BUR = SP/SA
19. b. Continuous-wave Doppler is transmitting 100% of the time, therefore the DF = 100%
20. c. SPL = λn, or wavelength times the number of cycles in the pulse
21. c. Phased array transducers operate by shocking the elements with minute time differences in between
22. a. If the power is reduced by half it is the same as a change of −3dB. Therefore, 18dB − 3dB = 15dB.
23. b. SPTP is the highest intensity, SATA is the lowest. Peaks are always higher than averages
24. c. Power is proportional to the amplitude squared. If the amplitude is increased threefold, the power increases by nine times
25. b. The average rate of attenuation in soft tissue is 0.7 dB/cm/MHz

26. c. The IRC and the ITC must total 100. If the ITC = 0.74, the IRC must equal 0.26

27. c. $Z = \rho c$, or impedance equals density times propagation speed

28. a. Rayleigh scattering occurs from reflectors that are significantly smaller than the wavelength of the incident beam, such as red blood cells

29. b. If the impedances of two media are identical, there cannot be reflection and there will be 100% transmission of sound

30. b. Total attenuation (dB) = ½ f × path length. Therefore (0.5 × 3.5) × 2 = 3.5 dB

31. b. The thinner the piezoelectric element, the higher the resonating frequency

32. c. The unit for impedance is Rayls

33. c. There can be no refraction when sound hits a reflector at 90° to the interface

34. a. ALARA stands for "As low as reasonably achievable"

35. a. Decibels (dB) represent the ratio between two parameters

36. c. Snell's law describes refraction at an interface

37. c. The attenuation coefficient in soft tissue is equal to one half of the frequency

38. b. ITC = 1 − IRC

39. b. The range equation ($d = ct/2$) provides the distance to the reflector

40. a. The attenuation coefficient (in dB/cm) in soft tissue is equal to one half of the frequency

41. c. To calculate distance to the reflector, the travel time and propagation speed must be known

42. a. Specular reflections occur when the interface (border) is larger than the incident wavelength

43. a. Use the reflection equation $I_r = I_i \times [(Z_2 - Z_1)/(Z_2 + Z_1)]^2$

44. d. The matching layer has an impedance between that of the piezoelectric element and the skin in order to improve transmission of sound into the patient

45. c. Quality factor = operating frequency/bandwidth

46. b. The piezoelectric effect occurs when electricity is applied and a pressure wave is generated

47. a. The transducer element in modern day transducers is a ceramic made up of lead zirconate titanate (PZT)

48. a. Diffraction occurs as a result of Huygen's principle and is a spreading of the wavefront

49. c. Ultrasound transducers must be cold sterilized

50. a. The thicker the element, the lower the frequency

51. c. Spatial resolution is the ability to discern two closely spaced reflectors as individual reflectors

52. a. Focusing improves lateral resolution and is unrelated to axial resolution

53. c. Bandwidth is the range of frequencies produced by the transducer

54. b. Decreasing the wavelength will increase the frequency, and thereby decrease divergence in the far field

55. a. The matching layer(s) impedance is chosen to improve the transmission of sound into the body

56. c. If the amount of damping decreases, the bandwidth decreases

57. b. The beam is smallest at the focal zone or focus
58. d. The near zone length is determined by both frequency and element diameter
59. c. The annular array has elements arranged into concentric rings
60. d. An increase of 10 dB is equal to a change of 10 times the initial intensity
61. c. The curvilinear (aka curved, convex) transducer has multiple elements on a curvature
62. c. Compensation is the same as TGC, or time gain compensation
63. b. The scan converter stores the echo information in memory before it is sent to the display
64. a. The pulser is responsible for producing the voltages that drive the transducer
65. a. The scan converter contains the analog-to-digital converter, memory, and digital-to-analog converter
66. d. The human eye has a dynamic range of about 20 dB and can discern 100 different shades of gray ranging from the lightest to the darkest
67. d. Most current ultrasound systems have 256 shades of gray
68. d. Shades of gray are 2^n, where n = the number of bits per pixel in memory. $2^4 = 16$
69. b. The transducer determines the spatial resolution of the system
70. c. The number 32 in binary is 100000
71. c. Preprocessing assigns received amplitudes to predetermined shades of gray
72. b. Compression is the opposite of dynamic range. Increasing the compression reduces the dynamic range
73. c. The unit for area is cm^2
74. a. Frequency and wavelength are inversely related
75. d. With tissue harmonic imaging (THI), there are decreased near-field artifacts
76. b. Infrasound is sound with a frequency less than 20 Hz
77. b. Audible sound is in the frequency range of 20 to 20,000 Hz
78. d. Pulse repetition frequency is changed by adjusting the depth
79. a. Period is the time it takes for one cycle to occur
80. d. Spatial pulse length is the length of the pulse
81. b. Since the propagation speed of medium 2 is less than the propagation speed of medium 1, the angle of transmission will be less than the angle of incidence ($\theta_2 < \theta_1$ if $C_2 < C_1$)
82. c. Propagation speed is only determined by the medium (specifically stiffness and density)
83. b. The slowest propagation speed of sound is through air
84. b. Intensity is a parameter that represents the strength of the beam
85. d. Pascal (Pa) is the unit for pressure amplitude
86. a. W/cm^2 is the unit of intensity
87. b. A change in amplitude will change the output power
88. d. Increasing output gain increases exposure to the patient
89. c. Increasing the power increases the intensity of the transmitted pulse
90. b. Intensity and power are directly proportional, so a doubling of the power causes a doubling of the intensity

91. a. Pulse repetition frequency is the number of pulses per second
92. c. Time is represented along the x-axis of the spectral waveform
93. b. The spatial pulse length is a distance, so meter (m) is the most correct answer
94. d. The hydrophone is used to test output intensity
95. c. Huygen's principle states that sound waves are the result of the interference of many wavelets produced as the face of the transducer
96. d. A-mode displays the amplitude of the reflectors along the y-axis
97. c. In B-mode imaging amplitude is the brightness of the dot, which is considered the z-axis of the image
98. c. Radial, or axial resolution, is determined by the spatial pulse length (SPL)
99. d. Decreasing the number of cycles in a pulse (n) or increasing the frequency (f) will improve the axial resolution
100. b. The axial resolution is one half of the SPL. Therefore, the axial resolution is 1.3 mm. Since the two reflectors are 1.3 mm apart, they will be resolved as two individual echoes
101. c. Divergence occurs in the far zone, or Fraunhofer zone
102. b. The larger the aperture, or element diameter, the longer the near zone
103. a. Resolution of two echoes parallel to the beam is the axial resolution
104. b. The more focal zones that are used, the worse the temporal resolution
105. a. The slice-thickness plane is focused with a lens in most modern transducers
106. a. If sound travels through a substance with a propagation speed less than 1540 m/s, the reflectors will be displayed too far away
107. d. A maximum temperature increase of 2°C appears to be safe
108. c. Both will travel at the same speed, that is to say that frequency and propagation speed are unrelated
109. c. An image that is purely black and white is called a bistable image
110. a. The bit, or binary digit, is the smallest unit of digital memory
111. d. In the Fresnel zone, or near zone, the beam area decreases with distance from the transducer
112. a. The receiver information is in analog form
113. b. Pixels can either be color or grayscale; they cannot be both at the same time
114. b. Write magnification enlarges the image before the image is stored in digital memory, thus preserving the pixel density
115. c. Amplitude and frequency are unrelated
116. a. The length of the pulse (SPL) and the pulse duration are directly related
117. c. Axial resolution does not vary with depth
118. a. If the pressure differential is increased, there is an increase in flow
119. b. This describes Poiseuille's law
120. c. Laminar flow is the most common type of flow in the body

Answer Key for Chapter Review Questions

CHAPTER 1

1. a. Stiffness is the ability of an object to resist compression and relates to the hardness of a medium.
2. a. An increase in pulse repetition period would lead to an increase in duty factor.
3. b. Bone, which has a propagation speed of 4080 m/s, has the highest propagation speed.
4. d. Lung tissue, which has a propagation speed 660 m/s, has the lowest propagation speed.
5. c. As imaging depth increases, the PRF decreases.
6. d. Refraction is a redirection of the transmitted sound beam. Snell's law describes the angle of transmission at an interface based on the angle of incidence and the propagation speeds of the two media.
7. b. Pressure is typically expressed in pascals.
8. b. The typical range of frequency for diagnostic ultrasound is 1 to 20 MHz.
9. a. The attenuation coefficient (in dB/cm) is the rate at which sound is attenuated per unit depth. It is equal to one half of the frequency ($f/2$) in soft tissue.
10. a. Micro denotes millionth.
11. d. Wavelength is distance over which one cycle occurs, or the distance from the beginning of one cycle to the end of the same cycle.
12. b. Stiffness and propagation speed are directly related: the stiffer the medium, the faster the propagation speed.
13. a. Areas of high pressure and density are referred to as compression.
14. c. Spatial pulse length equals the number of cycles in the pulse multiplied by the wavelength.
15. a. Density is typically measured in kilograms per centimeter cubed.
16. d. Attenuation is a decrease in the amplitude, power, and intensity of the sound beam as sound travels through tissue. There are three mechanisms of attenuation: absorption, reflection, and scattering.
17. b. The total amount of attenuation that occurs if a 6.0-MHz sound beam travels through 4 cm of soft tissue is 12 dB.
18. b. As imaging depth increases, the pulse repetition period increases.
19. b. If the pulse repetition frequency increases, the duty factor increases.
20. c. The duty factor is the percentage of time the ultrasound system is producing a sound.

21. a. Density and propagation speed are inversely related.
22. a. Power decreases as amplitude decreases.
23. b. Wavelength is equal to the propagation speed divided by the frequency.
24. d. Wavelength is determined by both the sound source and the medium.
25. c. Pulse repetition frequency is defined as the number of ultrasound pulses emitted in 1 second.
26. d. Pulse duration is only the active time or "on" time.
27. c. The inertia of a medium describes its density.
28. a. Frequency is determined by the sound source only.
29. b. "Centi" denotes hundredths.
30. b. The angle of transmission is greater than 40°.
31. c. Refraction is the change in direction of the transmitted sound beam that occurs with oblique incidence and dissimilar propagation speeds.
32. a. Propagation speed can be measured in millimeters per microsecond.
33. b. Absorption is the major component of attenuation.
34. d. In clinical imaging, the wavelengths measure between 0.1 and 0.8 mm.
35. b. The duty factor for continuous wave ultrasound is 100%.
36. b. Wavelength does not relate to the strength of the sound wave.
37. b. If power is decreased by half, intensity is decreased by half.
38. a. Damping of the sound beam decreases the spatial pulse length.
39. c. Axial resolution is the ability to resolve reflectors that lie parallel to the beam as distinct echoes.
40. a. The pulse repetition period is the time from the start of one pulse to the start of the next pulse, and therefore, it includes the "on" (or transmit) and "off" (or listening) times.
41. b. Pressure is measured in pascals or pounds per square inch.
42. c. Intensity is essentially equal to the power of a wave divided by the area over which the power is distributed.
43. c. Transducers have material within them that, when electronically stimulated, produces ultrasound waves. These materials most likely consist of some form of lead zirconate titanate.
44. d. If amplitude triples, then power increases by nine times.
45. b. Rarefaction is an area in the sound wave where the molecules are spread wider apart.
46. b. If only the density of the medium is increased, then the propagation speed will decrease.
47. d. Sound is technically a mechanical and longitudinal wave.
48. d. Amplitude is the maximum or minimum deviation of an acoustic variable from the average value of that variable.
49. c. 1 MHz is an ultrasonic frequency.
50. d. The average speed of sound in all soft tissue is considered to be 1540 m/s or 1.54 mm/μs.

CHAPTER 2

1. d. The focus is the narrowest part of the ultrasound beam.
2. c. The damping material, same as backing material, is the part of transducer assembly that reduces the number of cycles produced in a pulse.
3. c. The frame rate is determined by both the number of lines per frame and the imaging depth.
4. d. Temporal resolution, also known as frame rate, is the ability to display moving structures in real time.
5. b. The annular transducer utilizes elements arranged in concentric rings.
6. a. The curved linear array has a wider field of view compared with the phased array transducer.
7. d. The mechanical transducer does have moving parts.
8. b. Frequency, along with crystal diameter, determines the divergence in the far field.
9. a. An increase in line density would decrease temporal resolution.
10. d. Decreasing the imaging depth would increase the frame rate.
11. b. The diameter of the beam in the near zone (Fresnel zone) decreases.
12. a. Axial resolution is best in imaging.
13. c. A large crystal and high frequency would increase the near zone length.
14. c. A large crystal diameter and high frequency would decrease the beam divergence in the far field.
15. a. Imaging transducers have low quality factors and wide bandwidths.
16. b. Damping material decreases the spatial pulse length.
17. a. A curved pattern would produce focusing of the beam.
18. c. The focal point measures one half of the total beam width.
19. b. The matching layer is the component of the transducer that is used to step down the impedance from that of the element to that of the patient's skin.
20. b. The bandwidth is the range of frequencies within the sound beam.
21. a. Constructive interference occurs when in-phase waves meet and the amplitudes of the two waves are added to form one large wave.
22. c. The mechanical transducer utilizes a motor for beam steering.
23. a. The matching layer is composed of epoxy resin loaded with tungsten.
24. d. The linear sequenced array does not have elements arranged in a ring.
25. b. A smaller aperture results in a shorter near zone length.
26. c. Damping increases axial resolution.
27. a. Angular resolution is a synonym for lateral resolution.
28. b. Temporal resolution relates to the frame rate.
29. c. The far zone may also be referred to as the Fraunhofer zone.
30. d. Huygen's principle states that waves are the result of the interference of many wavelets produced at the face of the transducer.

31. b. Elevational resolution is the resolution in the third dimension of the beam, the slice-thickness plane.
32. a. The higher the frequency, the longer the near zone length.
33. c. Phasing is a method of focusing and/or steering the beam by applying electrical impulses to the piezoelectric elements with small time differences between shocks.
34. a. Spatial resolution consists of axial, elevational, and contrast resolution.
35. d. Annular array transducers are no longer used.
36. a. Continuous-wave transducers are not used for imaging.
37. b. The linear phased transducer is also referred to as a sector or vector transducer.
38. c. Backing material or the damping material of the transducer assembly reduces the number of cycles produced in a pulse.
39. b. The phased array produces a pie-shaped image.
40. b. The footprint is the part of the transducer that comes in contact with the patient.
41. d. Heat sterilization will kill pathogens but will unfortunately destroy the transducer as well.
42. a. Range resolution, also referred to as axial resolution, is the ability to accurately identify reflectors that are arranged parallel to the ultrasound beam.
43. c. Destructive interference occurs when out-of-phase waves meet. The amplitude of the resultant wave is smaller than either of the original waves.
44. a. A thinner piezoelectric element will yield a higher frequency.
45. d. At the face of the transducer, the beam diameter is equal to the element diameter.
46. c. The curved sequence array would be well suited for imaging abdominal structures.
47. a. The annular array transducer is not used to create 3D images.
48. b. The frame rate is equal to the pulse repetition frequency divided by the lines per frame.
49. a. Temporal resolution is the ability to represent structures in real time.
50. b. Ultrasound transducers are typically cold sterilized.

CHAPTER 3

1. b. The output gain is a pulser function. Changing it changes the intensity of the pulse.
2. b. Compensation adjusts for the attenuation of the beam, which causes echoes farther away from the transducer appear to be darker as the beam gets deeper.
3. b. Rectification is part of the "demodulation" component of the receiver.
4. b. The pixel, or picture element, is the smallest part of the image.
5. a. The bit, or binary digit, is the smallest amount of computer memory.

6. c. Rectification, part of demodulation, converts the negative component of the received signal into positive.

7. c. Bistable image is black and white with no other shades of gray.

8. d. Electrons are the negatively charged particles emitted by the electron gun of a CRT.

9. c. Magnetic deflector plates or coils steer the electrons.

10. b. In an interlaced image, such as with a CRT, there are two fields (odd and even) that make up one frame.

11. a. The number of shades of gray is equal to 2^n, where n = number of bits in memory (2^6 = 64 shades of gray).

12. b. The stronger the reflector, the brighter (whiter) the dot on the display.

13. a. The spatial detail of the display is improved with an increase in pixel density.

14. a. Slice thickness artifact is a result of too-wide an elevational (slice thickness) plane.

15. b. Enhancement occurs behind a weak attenuator like fluid or a cyst.

16. a. Output power is controlled by the pulser.

17. d. Reject (threshold) removes unwanted noise from the signal by eliminating echoes below a certain threshold.

18. c. Compression is the opposite of dynamic range, which is the range of echoes in a signal. Increasing the compression decreases the dynamic range.

19. b. Mirror-image artifact occurs as a result of sound refracting off of a strong reflector, causing a duplicate object to appear on the other side of the strong reflector.

20. d. $d = ct/2$. To compute the distance to the reflector, you need to know the round-trip time and the propagation speed of the medium. Assuming soft tissue, $d = 0.77t$ where "d" is the depth of the reflector and "t" represents the round-trip time of the pulse.

21. a. Contrast resolution is the ability to discern different shades of gray from each other.

22. b. Postprocessing, a function of the digital-to-analog converter, gets the signal ready for the display.

23. b. In B-mode, or brightness mode imaging, the brightness of the dot corresponds to the strength of the reflector.

24. c. M-mode, or motion mode imaging, displays movement of the reflectors as they occur along one scan line.

25. d. Time is along the x-axis of an M-mode image with depth along the y-axis.

26. b. The patient produces the harmonic signal that is received by the transducer.

27. a. In tissue harmonic imaging, the fundamental (transmitted) frequency is filtered out of the received signal and only the harmonic signal produced by the patient is displayed.

28. d. The range equation is $d = 0.77t$, where t is the round-trip time. Only the time to the reflector is given, not the round-trip time. Therefore, the given time must be doubled to 52 μs ($d = 0.77(52) = 40$ mm, or 4 cm).

29. c. Rewrite the range equation to solve for time ($T = d/0.77$) ($T = 20/0.77 = 26$ μs).

30. d. Subdicing, tissue harmonics, and apodization are all methods used to reduce or eliminate grating lobes.

31. a. The beam former determines the strength, or amplitude, of the voltage pulses.

32. c. Coded excitation improves the signal-to-noise ratio of the image, in that there is less noise.

33. b. Increasing the gain is the preferred way of brightening the image. Increasing the output (power) should be the last choice.

34. a. Read zoom is a postprocessing function, and therefore occurs in the D-to-A converter.

35. c. Write zoom is the higher-quality zoom because it preserves the pixel density. It is a preprocessing function, and therefore the image must be live.

36. d. Compensation, or TGC (time gain compensation) is needed to brighten the echoes that are diminished as a result of attenuation.

37. c. The voxel, or volume element, is the smallest component of a 3D image.

38. b. Fill-in interpolation is needed when there are gaps between scan lines. The machines make up (guesses) what pixels should be placed in between the scan lines based on the shades of gray along the actual scan lines.

39. c. VHS (abbreviation for Video Home System) uses a magnetic tape to store images.

40. a. Reverberation occurs when sound bounces between two strong reflectors.

41. d. Grating lobes occurs when sound energy is produced off of the main axis of the beam.

42. a. When the actual propagation speed is greater than 1540 m/s, the reflector will be placed too close to the transducer.

43. b. Shadows are formed from sounds traveling through strongly attenuating areas.

44. d. Echo information goes from the memory to the digital-to-analog converter to be processed for display and archiving.

45. a. A-mode, or amplitude mode, is still used in ophthalmology imaging.

46. a. The receiver does not affect the amount of sound entering the patient.

47. c. $2^1 = 2$ shades of gray, or bistable (black and white).

48. c. The master synchronizer pays attention to the timing of the pulses.

49. b. Frequency compounding improves contrast resolution and reduces speckle by imaging with multiple frequencies and averaging them out.

50. d. The machine always assumes 1540 m/s, which may be a cause of artifact.

CHAPTER 4

1. c. The heart provides the potential energy at the beginning of the cardiovascular system.

2. d. Hydrostatic pressure is pressure from gravity.

3. a. Plug flow occurs in large vessels (e.g., aorta) and at the entrance of vessels.

4. b. When the scale (PRF) setting is increased, the Nyquist limit is increased, thereby decreasing the likelihood of aliasing.

5. a. The frequency of CW transducers is determined by the oscillator frequency.

6. c. The Doppler shift is highest when the beam is parallel to flow (i.e., at a 0° angle).

7. d. To eliminate aliasing the frequency shift needs to be decreased.

8. a. The frequency of the reflected sound increases as sound moves toward the transducer.

9. a. The higher the pressure difference, the greater the amount of flow.

10. c. Amplitude is not part of the Doppler equation.

11. a. Voltage (pressure difference) = Current (flow) × Resistance.

12. c. A Reynolds number > 2000 indicates turbulence.

13. b. Q = VA. As the area increases, the velocity decreases in order to maintain the flow as a constant.

14. c. The calf muscle pump, inspiration, and venous valves all aid in the return of venous blood to the heart.

15. a. Gravity causes the highest pressure to be in the feet of an erect patient.

16. b. A 75% decrease in area is equivalent to a 50% decrease in diameter.

17. b. Exercise in a normal patient causes vasodilatation, which causes decreased peripheral resistance.

18. c. If there is no reflector motion, the reflected frequency equals the incident frequency.

19. b. The higher the frequency, the greater the intensity of the scatter.

20. a. An increase in the Doppler angle causes a decrease in the frequency shift because the frequency shift is calculated based on the cosine of the angle, not the angle itself.

21. d. Phase quadrature is the processing technique used to detect positive versus negative frequency shifts.

22. b. Two piezoelectric elements are needed for a CW device. One element continuously sends and the other continuously receives.

23. c. Aliasing occurs when the signal is not sampled often enough.

24. d. Fast Fourier transform (FFT) is the signal processing technique used for spectral Doppler.

25. c. The RI = PSV − EDV/PSV.

26. a. The spectral amplitude is proportional to the number of red blood cells present within the signal.

27. a. Spectral broadening is a widening of the envelope of the spectral Doppler waveform and appears as a filling-in of the spectral window.

28. b. The sweep speed adjusts the number of waveforms that appear on the spectral display at one time.

29. c. When the spectral gain is too high, the velocities may be overmeasured.

30. d. At a 90° angle to flow the Doppler shift is zero.

31. c. Autocorrelation is the signal processing technique used for color Doppler imaging.

32. b. Only one crystal or active element is needed for PW Doppler.

33. b. Power Doppler uses the strength, or amplitude, of the frequency shift.
34. b. In triplex mode, the spectral waveform is displayed simultaneously with the color and 2D image.
35. a. The duty factor, or percentage of time the sound is being transmitted, of a CW beam is 1 or 100%.
36. c. CW beams have a large sample volume that may sample several vessels at once.
37. b. Color Doppler has very poor temporal resolution (slow frame rates).
38. a. Color Doppler is a PW technique, and therefore has the same limitation on PRF as spectral Doppler.
39. c. Aliasing occurs at a frequency shift greater than ½ PRF. If the PRF is 5000 Hz, then the Nyquist limit is 2500 Hz, or 2.5 kHz. Therefore, any frequency shift more than 2.5 kHz would exhibit aliasing.
40. d. The frequency shift is typically 1/1000th of the operating frequency, which is in the audible range of sound (20 to 20,000 Hz).
41. c. The typical ensemble length is 10 to 20 pulses per scan line, although it may be as low as 3.
42. a. Laminar flow has its highest velocities in the center of the vessel.
43. d. Color Doppler imaging cannot measure peak systolic or end diastolic velocities, only mean velocities.
44. b. Power Doppler is obtained by measuring the amplitude of the Doppler shift.
45. c. According to Bernoulli, in a region of narrowing there is an increase in the velocity of the blood along with a corresponding decrease in pressure.
46. d. In the presence of turbulence, there is spectral broadening, a vertical thickening of the spectral envelope.
47. c. The pressure of the inside of a vessel compared to the outside pressure is its transmural pressure.
48. b. A delay in the upstroke of an arterial waveform, or tardus parvus waveform, is indicative of proximal obstruction.
49. c. The wall filter control eliminates the low frequency shift component of the spectral waveform.
50. a. Monophasic flow is seen proximal to a low-resistance bed.

CHAPTER 5

1. b. Comprehensive maintenance should be performed at least semiannually.
2. d. The Doppler phantom uses a moving belt, vibrating string or a fluid pump to simulate fluid moving through the body.
3. c. The AIUM test object cannot evaluate contrast resolution.
4. b. Vertical depth calibration evaluates the distance from the transducer or the depth of reflectors.
5. d. The report of malfunctioning equipment should be done immediately.
6. d. Cardiovascular Credential International (CCI) offers certification exams in cardiac and vascular testing.

7. b. Accreditation, or lab accreditation, is a voluntary process that acknowledges an organization's competency and credibility according to standards and essentials set forth by a reliable source.

8. c. Sensitivity is the ability of a system to display low-level echoes.

9. c. Slice-thickness errors will cause artificial echoes to appear within a cystic structure.

10. a. Vertical distance indicates the maximum depth of visualization.

11. c. Preventative maintenance is a methodical way of evaluating equipment's performance on a routine basis to ensure proper and accurate equipment function.

12. d. The sonographer plays a vital role in the maintenance of equipment and quality of care.

13. c. Axial resolution is the ability to accurately identify reflectors that are arranged front to back and parallel to the ultrasound beam.

14. c. The tissue-equivalent phantom's integrity must be maintained, as the container must be airtight to avoid degradation of the tissue properties inside the phantom. Also, the storage area temperature should also be monitored in order to preserve the acoustic properties of the phantom.

15. d. The slice-thickness phantom is test object that evaluates the elevation resolution, or the thickness portion, of the sound beam perpendicular to the imaging plane.

16. a. The AIUM test object is an outdated test object that used an acrylic tank that was filled with fluid; the fluid in this test object attempted to simulate the speed of sound in soft tissue.

17. c. The test object that mimics the acoustic properties of human tissue and is used to ensure proper equipment performance is the tissue-equivalent phantom.

18. b. Doppler test objects are used to evaluate the flow direction, the depth capability or penetration of the Doppler beam, and the accuracy of sample volume location and measured velocity.

19. b. The American Registry of Diagnostic Medical Sonography is not an accreditation body.

20. d. The American Institute of Ultrasound in Medicine is not a certification granting body.

CHAPTER 6

1. c. The American Institute of Ultrasound in Medicine (AIUM) formed and suggests the utilization of the ALARA principle: As Low As Reasonably Achievable. This term relates the amount of exposure time for the sonographer and the patient during a diagnostic ultrasound examination.

2. b. Verifying the patient's wristband information for identifying markers, which includes the patient's name, medical record number, and date of birth, is an essential part of patient care.

3. c. If a patient does not speak English, or national language, the sonographer should obtain an interpreter. This practice will ensure that the patient is completely informed about the procedure prior to the procedure taking place.

4. a. Hyperglycemic hyperosmolar nonketotic syndrome is a diabetic syndrome characterized by excessive urination and dehydration.

5. b. Shock is the body's pathologic response to illness, trauma, or severe physiologic or emotional stress.

6. a. The classic presentation of cardiac arrest includes a loss of consciousness, loss of blood pressure, dilation of the pupils, and possibly seizures.

7. c. Hand washing is the most effective way to prevent the spread of infection.

8. b. Cavitation is the action of an acoustic field within a fluid to generate bubbles. There are two types of cavitation: stable and transient. Stable cavitation produces bubbles that oscillate, or fluctuate, in size but do not rupture. Transient cavitation, also referred to as collapse, has the potential of causing the most biologic damage.

9. a. Streaming is when acoustic fields cause motion of fluids.

10. d. The thermal index is the calculation used to predict the maximum temperature elevation in tissues as a result of attenuation of sound.

11. b. The maximum heating of tissue is related to the sound beams spatial pulse temporal average (SPTA).

12. d. HIPAA does not attempt to deal with safe practices or cleanliness in the health care setting.

13. c. Radiation forces are exerted by a sound beam on an absorber or reflector that can alter structures.

14. c. Transient cavitation, also referred to as collapse, has the potential of causing the most biologic damage. With transient cavitation, larger bubbles are produced and subsequently rupture. The rupture of these bubbles produces a shock wave and an increase in tissue temperature in that area. This increase in temperature has been associated with biologic effects.

15. b. The mechanical index was developed to assist in evaluating the likelihood of cavitation to occur.

16. d. Cardiogenic shock is failure of the heart to pump the proper amount of blood to the vital organs. It can be caused by myocardial infarction, cardiac tamponade, dysrhythmias, or other cardiac pathology.

17. a. A nosocomial infection is best described as a hospital-acquired infection.

18. c. Anaphylactic shock is a subcategory of distributive shock that results from an exaggerated allergic reaction, leading to vasodilation and pooling in the peripheral blood vessels. It can be caused by medications, iodinated contrast agents that are often used in x-ray procedures, and insect venoms.

19. c. A urinary tract infection is a common infection acquired during a hospital stay.

20. d. A reservoir is needed for an infectious agent to initially survive.

21. d. Hepatitis B and C viruses, human immunodeficiency virus (HIV), tuberculosis (TB), and methicillin-resistant *Staphylococcus aureus* (MRSA) are among the list of communicable diseases that may be transmitted in the hospital from a patient to a health care worker.

22. c. Needles would be considered a means of transmission.

23. a. These precautions deal with safety measures that should apply to blood, all body fluids, secretions, excretions, nonintact skin, and mucous membranes. Sweat is not included.

24. d. Image orientation does not have to be removed from the image.

25. c. Tuberculosis is an airborne disease found in the lungs, and possibly other organs, of an infected person. The TB bacteria are released from an infected individual most often when that person coughs, sneezes, speaks, or sings.

26. a. Most staff infections manifest as an infected area on the skin.

27. a. Hepatitis is inflammation of the liver.

28. d. Nonthermal mechanisms include radiation forces, streaming, and acoustic cavitation, with the most worrisome being the later.

29. d. The primary reason why tissue heats as sound is attenuated in the human body is absorption.

30. a. No effects have been observed for an unfocused beam having free-field SPTA intensities below 100 mW/cm².

31. d. Obstructive shock results from pathologic conditions that interfere with the normal pumping action of the heart. It can be caused by pulmonary embolism, pulmonary hypertension, arterial stenosis, and possibly tumors that obstruct normal blood flow to the heart.

32. b. Diabetic ketoacidosis occurs when a patient has insufficient insulin, resulting in excess glucose production by the liver. The patient may have sweet smelling breath.

33. a. In tissues that contain well-defined gas bodies, for example, lung, no effects have been observed for in situ peak rarefactional pressures below approximately 0.4 MPa or mechanical index values less than approximately 0.4.

34. c. No effects have been observed for an unfocused beam having free-field SPTA intensities below 100 mW/cm², or a focused beam having intensities below 1 W/cm², or thermal index values of less than 2.

35. b. A portal of exit from the reservoir must be available for the pathogen to be transmitted to another individual.

36. a. The TB bacteria are released from an infected individual most often when that person coughs, sneezes, speaks, or sings.

37. d. Complications of diabetes include tachycardia, headache, blurred vision, extreme thirst, polyuria, or a sweet odor to the breath (in diabetic ketoacidosis).

38. b. HIV is not spread through kissing.

39. d. The compensatory patient will experience cold and clammy skin, decreased urine output, increased respiration, reduced bowel sounds, and increased anxiety. If shock is allowed to progress, the patient's blood pressure will drop, their respirations will decrease, and they will experience tachycardia, chest pain, and possibly have a loss of mental alertness.

40. a. Alcohol-based hand rubs should never take the place of proper hand washing.

41. c. The carotid pulse should be evaluated in the nonresponsive patient.

42. b. Glutaraldehyde-based solutions may be used to sterilize sonographic equipment, not act as personal protective equipment.

43. d. Barrier techniques can be used to prevent the spread of infection. These methods include sterilization, decontamination, and disposing of infected waste.

44. c. An accidental needle stick would be the most likely means of transmission of HIV from a patient to a sonographer.

45. d. Tuberculosis is an airborne disease.

46. b. Nonthermal mechanisms may also be referred to as mechanical mechanisms.

47. c. There are three types of distributive shocks: neurogenic, septic, and anaphylactic.

48. a. No independently confirmed adverse effects caused by exposure from present diagnostic ultrasound instruments have been reported in human patients in the absence of contrast agents.

49. b. The use of gloves should never replace proper hand washing.

50. d. Transient cavitation, also referred to as collapse, has the potential of causing the most biologic damage. With transient cavitation, larger bubbles are produced and subsequently rupture.

Glossary

13 μs rule—the rule that states that it takes 13 μs for sound to travel 1 cm in soft tissue

absorption—the conversion of sound energy to heat

acoustic cavitation—the production of bubbles in a liquid medium

acoustic speckle—the interference pattern caused by scatterers that produces the granular appearance of tissue on a sonographic image

AIUM test object—an outdated test object that used an acrylic tank that was filled with fluid; the fluid in this test object attempted to simulate the speed of sound in soft tissue

ALARA—as low as reasonably achievable; the principle that states one should always use the lowest power and shortest scanning time possible to reduce potential exposure to the patient

aliasing—the wraparound of the spectral or color Doppler display that occurs when the frequency shift exceeds the Nyquist limit; only occurs with pulsed-wave Doppler

A-mode—amplitude mode; the height of the spike on the image is related to the strength (amplitude) of the echo generated by the reflector

amplification—the part of the receiver that increases or decreases the received echoes equally, regardless of depth

amplitude—the maximum or minimum deviation of an acoustic variable from the average value of that variable; the strength of the reflector

amplitude mode—*see* key term A-mode

analog-to-digital (A-to-D) converter—the part of the digital scan converter that converts the analog signals from the receiver to binary for processing by the computer

anechoic—without echoes, or black

angle correct—the tool used to inform the machine what the flow angle is so that velocities can be accurately calculated

aperture—the diameter of the piezoelectric element(s) producing the beam

apodization—the technique that varies the voltage to the individual elements to reduce grating lobes

array—the transducer with multiple active elements

artifacts—echoes on the screen that are not representative of actual anatomy, or reflectors in the body that are not displayed on the screen

attenuation—a decrease in the amplitude, power, and intensity of the sound beam as sound travels through tissue

attenuation coefficient—the rate at which sound is attenuated per unit depth

autocorrelation—the color Doppler processing technique that assesses pixels as stationary or in motion

automatic external defibrillator—a portable device that is used to detect and treat abnormal heart rhythms with electrical defibrillation

automatic scanning—same as real-time ultrasound

axial resolution—the ability to accurately identify reflectors that are arranged parallel to the ultrasound beam

backing material—the damping material of the transducer assembly, which reduces the number of cycles produced in a pulse

backscatter—scattered sound waves that make their way back to the transducer and produce an image on the display

bandwidth—the range of frequencies present within the beam

BART—acronym used in echocardiography describing color Doppler scale: "*blue away, red toward*"

baseline—the operator-adjustable dividing line between positive frequency shifts and negative frequency shifts on spectral and color Doppler

beam former—the instrument that shapes and steers the beam on the transmit end

Bernoulli's principle—the principle that describes the inverse relationship between velocity and pressure

bidirectional Doppler—the Doppler device that can detect positive and negative Doppler shifts

binary—the digital language of zeroes and ones

bistable—black-and-white image

bit—the smallest unit of memory in a digital device

B-mode—brightness mode; the brightness of the dots is proportional to the strength of the echo generated by reflector

boundary layer—the stationary layer of blood cells immediately adjacent to the vessel wall

brightness—the term describing the intensity or luminance of the color Doppler display

brightness mode—*see* key term B-mode

byte—eight bits of memory

calf muscle pump—the muscles in the calf that, upon contraction, propel venous blood toward the heart

cathode ray tube (CRT)—display that uses an electron gun to produce a stream of electrons toward a phosphor-coated screen

clutter—acoustic noise in the color and/or spectral Doppler signal

coded excitation—a way of processing the pulse to improve contrast resolution and reduce speckle

color Doppler imaging (CDI)—Doppler shift information presented as a color (hue) superimposed over the grayscale image

color priority—the setting for color Doppler that allows the operator to select frequency shift threshold; it determines whether color pixels should be displayed preferentially over grayscale pixels

comet tail—a type of reverberation artifact caused by small reflectors (i.e., surgical clips)

compensation—the function of the receiver that changes the brightness of the echo amplitudes to compensate for attenuation with depth

compression (receiver function)—the function of the receiver that decreases the range of signal amplitudes present with the machine's receiver; opposite of dynamic range

compression (sound wave)—an area in the sound wave where the molecules are pushed closer together

constructive interference—occurs when in-phase waves meet; the amplitudes of the two waves are added to form one large wave

continuity equation—the equation that describes the change in velocity as the area changes in order to maintain the volume of blood flow ($Q = VA$)

continuous wave—sound that is continuously transmitted

continuous-wave (CW) Doppler—Doppler device that uses continuous-wave ultrasound transmission

contrast resolution—the ability to differentiate one shade of gray from another

critical stenosis—the point at which a stenosis is hemodynamically significant with a pressure drop distal to the stenosis

crystal—a synonym for the active element of the transducer, the piezoelectric part of the transducer assembly that produces sound

Curie point—the temperature at which an ultrasound transducer will gain its piezoelectric properties, and also the temperature at which a transducer will lose the ability to produce sound if heated again above this temperature

curved sequenced array—the transducer commonly referred to as curvilinear or convex probe

damping—the process of reducing the number of cycles of each pulse in order to improve axial resolution

damping material—same as backing material, the part of transducer assembly that reduces the number of cycles produced in a pulse

decibels (dB)—a unit that establishes a relationship or comparison between two values of power or intensity

demodulation—the function of the receiver that makes the signal easier to process by performing rectification and smoothing

density—mass per unit volume

depth ambiguity—the inability to determine the depth of the reflector if the pulses are sent out too fast for them to be timed

destructive interference—occurs when out-of-phase waves meet; the amplitude of the resultant wave is smaller than either of the original waves

diabetes mellitus—a group of metabolic diseases that result from a chronic disorder of carbohydrate metabolism

diabetic ketoacidosis—a complication of diabetes that results from a severe lack of insulin

diastole—the relaxation of the heart following contraction

diffraction—spreading of the beam that occurs after the focal zone

digital-to-analog (D-to-A) converter—part of the digital scan converter that converts the binary signals from computer memory to analog for display and storage

directional power Doppler—combination of color Doppler and power Doppler that provides the sensitivity of power Doppler with color Doppler's ability to provide for direction of blood flow

directly related—relationship that implies that if one variable decreases, the other also decreases or if one variable increases, the other also increases

distance—how far apart objects are

divergence—spreading of the beam that occurs in the far zone

Doppler effect—the change in the frequency of the received signal related to motion of reflector

Doppler equation—the equation that explains the relationship of the Doppler frequency shift (F_D) to the frequency of the transducer (f), the velocity of the blood (v), the angle to blood flow ($\cos \theta$), and the propagation speed (c)

Doppler phantom—the test object used to evaluate the flow direction, the depth capability or penetration of the Doppler beam, and the accuracy of sample volume location and measured velocity

duplex—the real-time 2D imaging combined with the spectral Doppler display

duty factor—the percentage of time that sound is actually being produced

dynamic range—the series of echo amplitudes present within the signal

edge shadowing—refraction artifact caused by the curved surface of reflector

elasticity—*see* key term stiffness

electrical interference—arc-like bands that occur when the machine is too close to an unshielded electrical device

element—the piezoelectric part of the transducer assembly that produces sound

elevation plane—*see* key term slice-thickness plane

elevational resolution—the resolution in the third dimension of the beam, the slice-thickness plane

energy gradient—the difference in energy between two points ($E_1 - E_2$)

enhancement—an artifact caused by sound passing through area of lower attenuation

ensemble length—the number of pulses per scan line in color Doppler; also referred to as "packet size"

far zone—the diverging part of the beam distal to the focal point

Fast Fourier transform (FFT)—a mathematical process used for analyzing and processing the Doppler signal to produce the spectral waveform

field—one half of a frame on the display

fill-in interpolation—places pixels where there is no signal information based on adjacent scan lines

flash artifact—a motion artifact caused by the movement of tissue when using power Doppler

flow—the volume of blood per unit time; typically measured in L/min or mL/s; represented by the symbol Q

focal point—the area of the beam with the smallest beam diameter

footprint—the portion of the transducer that is in contact with the patient's skin

frame—one complete ultrasound image

frame rate—the number of frames per second

Fraunhofer zone—*see* key term far zone

frequency—the number of cycles per second

frequency compounding—averages the frequencies across the image to improve contrast resolution and reduce speckle

frequency shift—the difference between the transmitted and received frequencies

Fresnel zone—*see* key term near zone

friction—a form of resistance; caused by two materials rubbing against each other, thereby converting energy to heat

fundamental frequency—the operating or resonating frequency emitted by the transducer

grating lobes—an artifact caused by extraneous sound not along primary beam path; occurs with arrays; reduced or eliminated by apodization, subdicing, and tissue harmonics

gravitational potential energy—describes the relationship between gravity, density of the blood, and distance between an arbitrary reference point; also known as "hydrostatic pressure"

grayscale test objects—the testing phantoms that allow the evaluation of an ultrasound machine's ability to test grayscale sensitivity (contrast resolution) using various transducer frequencies

Health Insurance Portability and Accountability Act—the Act enacted in 1996 by the United States Congress, which, among many goals, upholds patient confidentiality and the use of electronic medical records

hemodynamics—the study of blood flow through the blood vessels of the body

hepatitis—inflammation of the liver

horizontal calibration—the ability to place echoes in the proper location horizontally and perpendicular to the sound beam

hue—a term used to describe displayed colors (e.g., red, blue, green)

Huygen's principle—states that waves are the result of the interference of many wavelets produced at the face of the transducer

hydrophone—a device used to measure output intensity of the transducer

hydrostatic pressure—*see* key term gravitational potential energy

hyperechoic—displayed echoes that are relatively brighter than the surrounding tissue; may also be referred to as echogenic

hyperglycemic hyperosmolar nonketotic syndrome—a diabetic syndrome characterized by excessive urination and dehydration

hypoechoic—displayed echoes that are relatively darker than the surrounding tissue

hypoglycemia—a lower-than-normal blood sugar level

impedance—the resistance to the propagation of sound through a medium

inertia—Newton's principle that states that an object at rest stays at rest and an object in motion stays in motion, unless acted on by an outside force

innervated—supplied with nerves

in-phase—waves whose peaks and troughs overlap

intensity—the power of the wave divided by the area over which it is spread; the energy per unit area

intensity reflection coefficient—the percentage of sound reflected at an interface

intensity transmission coefficient—the percentage of sound transmitted at an interface

interface—the dividing line between two different media

inversely related—relationship that implies that if one variable decreases, the other increases or if one variable increases, the other decreases

kinetic energy—the energy form of flowing blood

lab accreditation—a voluntary process that acknowledges an organization's competency and credibility according to standards and essentials set forth by a reliable source

laminar flow—the flow profile represented by blood that travels in nonmixing layers of different velocities, with the fastest flow in the center and the slowest flow near the vessel walls

lateral resolution—the ability to accurately identify reflectors that are arranged perpendicular to the ultrasound beam

law of conservation of energy—the total amount of energy in a system never changes, although it might be in a different form from which it started

lead zirconate titanate—abbreviated as PZT, this is the man-made ceramic of which many transducer elements are made

linear phased array—the transducer that uses phasing, or small time differences, to steer and focus the beam

linear sequenced array—the transducer commonly referred to as a "linear probe"

liquid crystal display (LCD)—display that uses the twisting and untwisting of liquid crystals in front of a light source

longitudinal waves—the molecules of the medium vibrate back and forth in the same direction that the wave is traveling

luminance—the brightness of the color Doppler image

master synchronizer—the timing component of the ultrasound machine that notes how long it takes for signals to return from reflectors (*see* key term range equation)

matching layer—the component of the transducer that is used to step down the impedance from that of the element to that of the patient's skin

mechanical index—the calculation used to assist in evaluating the likelihood of cavitation to occur

mechanical scanheads—transducers with a motor for steering the beam

medium—any form of matter: solid, liquid, or gas

mirror image—an artifact caused by sound bouncing off of strong reflector and causing a structure to appear on both sides of the reflector

mm Hg—millimeters of mercury

M-mode—motion mode; used to display motion of the reflectors

motion mode—*see* key term M-mode

multipath—an artifact caused by the beam bouncing off of several reflectors before returning to the transducer

near zone length—the length of the region from the transducer face to the focal point

near zone—the part of the beam between the element and the focal point

noise—low-level echoes on the display that do not contribute useful diagnostic information

nondirectional Doppler—Doppler device that cannot differentiate between positive and negative frequency shifts

nonlinear propagation—principle that pressure waves change in shape as they travel deeper, though in a disproportionate way

nonsinusoidal—waves that are not pure sine waves

nonspecular reflectors—reflectors that are smaller than the wavelength of the incident beam

normal incidence—angle of incidence is 90° to the interface

nosocomial infection—a hospital-acquired infection

Nyquist limit—the maximum frequency shift sampled without aliasing; equal to one half the pulse repetition frequency

oblique incidence—angle of incidence is lesser than or greater than 90° to the interface

Ohm's law—a law used in electronics in which flow is equal to the pressure differential divided by resistance

oscillator—the component of a continuous-wave Doppler device that produces the voltage that drives the transducer

out-of-phase—waves that are 180° opposite each other; the peak of one wave overlaps the trough of the other and vice versa

output—output power; strength of sound entering the patient

overall gain—receiver function that increases or decreases all the echo amplitudes equally

packet size—the number of pulses per scan line; also called ensemble length

PACS—Picture Archiving and Communication System; a type of display and storage device commonly used in ultrasound and other imaging modalities

parameter—a measurable quantity

particle motion—the movement of molecules due to propagating sound energy

path length—distance to the reflector

period—the time it takes for one cycle to occur

persistence—the averaging of color frames in order to display blood flow with a low signal-to-noise ratio

phase quadrature—the component of the Doppler device that determines positive opposed to negative frequency shifts and, therefore, direction of blood flow

phasic flow—the characteristic waveform of peripheral veins; flow is determined by respiratory variations as a result of intrathoracic pressure changes

phasicity—in arteries, the phasicity describes shape of the waveform based on the resistiveness of the distal bed (e.g., triphasic, biphasic, monophasic). In veins, phasicity describes the flow pattern that results from respiratory variation

phasing—the method of focusing and/or steering the beam by applying electrical impulses to the piezoelectric elements with small time differences between shocks

piezoelectric—the ability to convert pressure into electricity and electricity into pressure

piezoelectric materials—a material that generates electricity when pressure is applied to it, and one that changes shape when electricity is applied to it; also referred to as the element

pixel (picture element)—the smallest component of a 2D digital image

plug flow—the flow profile represented by blood typically flowing at the same velocity

Poiseuille's law—the law that describes the relationship of resistance, pressure, and flow

postprocessing—occurs in the D-to-A converter; the image must be frozen

potential energy—pressure energy created by the beating heart

power—the rate at which work is performed or energy is transmitted

power Doppler—amplitude mode of Doppler where it is not the shift itself that provides the signal, but the strength (amplitude) of the shift; amplitude is directly proportional to the number of red blood cells

preprocessing—occurs in the A-to-D converter; the image must be live

pressure—force per unit area or the concentration of force

pressure gradient—the difference between pressures at two ends of a blood vessel

preventative maintenance—a methodical way of evaluating equipment's performance on a routine basis to ensure proper and accurate equipment function

propagate—to transmit through a medium

propagation speed—the speed at which a sound wave travels through a medium

pulsatility—blood that flows in a pattern representative of the beating heart, with increases and decreases in pressure and blood flow velocity

pulse duration—the time during which the sound is actually being transmitted; the "on" time

pulse repetition frequency—the number of pulses of sound produced in 1 second

pulse repetition period—the time taken for a pulse to occur

pulsed wave—sound that is sent out in pulses

pulsed-wave (PW) Doppler—the Doppler technique that uses pulses of sound to obtain Doppler signals from a user-specified depth

pulser—part of the beam former that controls the amount of energy in the pulse

quality assurance program—a planned program consisting of scheduled equipment-testing activities that confirm correct performance of equipment

quality factor (Q-factor)—the operating frequency of the transducer divided by the bandwidth

radiation forces—forces exerted by a sound beam on an absorber or reflector that can alter structures

range equation—equation used to calculate the distance to the reflector; in soft tissue, $d = 0.77t$ where "d" is the depth of the reflector and "t" represents the round-trip time of the pulse

range gate—the gate placed by the operator in the region where Doppler sampling is desired; used with pulsed-wave Doppler

range resolution—the ability to determine the depth of echoes by timing how long it takes for the echoes to go from the transducer to the reflector and back; utilized by pulsed-wave devices

rarefaction—an area in the sound wave where the molecules are spread wider apart

Rayleigh scatterers—very small reflectors

read zoom—the type of magnification performed in the D-to-A converter (postprocessing) that magnifies the image by enlarging the pixels

real-time—live ultrasound, also known as "automatic scanning"

receiver—the component of the machine that processes the signals coming back from the patient

rectification—the part of the receiver that inverts the negative voltages to positives

reflection—the echo; part of sound that returns from an interface

refraction—change in direction of the transmitted sound beam that occurs with oblique incidence and dissimilar propagation speeds

registration—the ability to place echoes in the correct location

rejection—function of the receiver that is used to reduce image noise; sets a threshold below which the signal will not be displayed

resistance—the downstream impedance to flow; determined by vessel length, vessel radius, and viscosity of blood

reverberation—an artifact caused by the beam bouncing between two strong reflectors

Reynolds number—the formula used to quantitate the presence of turbulence; Reynolds numbers greater than 2000 typically indicate turbulence

ring-down—a type of reverberation artifact caused by air

sample volume—the area within the range gate where the Doppler signals are obtained

saturation—the amount of white added to a hue; the more white there is, the less saturated the color

scale—the spectral Doppler and color Doppler tool that controls the number of pulses transmitted per second to obtain the Doppler information; also known as pulse repetition in spectral Doppler and color Doppler

scan converter—the part of the ultrasound machine that processes the signals from the receiver; consists of the A-to-D converter, computer memory, and D-to-A converter

scan line—created when one or more pulses of sound return from the tissue containing information related to the depth and amplitude of the reflectors

scattering—the phenomenon that occurs when sound waves are forced to deviate from a straight path secondary to changes within the medium

section-thickness plane—*see* slice-thickness plane

sensitivity—the ability of a system to display low-level or weak echoes

shadowing—an artifact caused by the failure of sound to pass through a strong attenuator

shock—the body's pathologic response to illness, trauma, or severe physiologic or emotional stress

shock excitation—applying electrical energy to the piezoelectric element causes it to resonate

side lobes—an artifact caused by extraneous sound that is not found along the primary beam path; occurs with single-element transducers

slice-thickness phantom—the test object that evaluates the elevation resolution, or the thickness portion, of the sound beam perpendicular to the imaging plane

slice-thickness plane—the third dimension of the beam

smoothing—part of the demodulation component of the receiver; an "envelope" is wrapped around the signal to eliminate the "humps"

Snell's law—used to describe the angle of transmission at an interface based on the angle of incidence and the propagation speeds of the two media

sound—a traveling variation in pressure

spatial pulse length—the length of a pulse

spatial resolution—refers to axial, lateral, contrast, and elevational resolution

speckle reduction—algorithm used in signal processing to reduce the amount of acoustic speckle

spectral broadening—the filling of the spectral window

spectral window—the area underneath the envelope on the spectral display

specular reflections—reflections that occur when the sound impinges upon a large, smooth reflector at a 90° angle

stenosis—pathologic narrowing of a blood vessel

stiffness—the ability of an object to resist compression and relates to the hardness of a medium

streaming—when acoustic fields cause motion of fluids

subdicing—dividing the piezoelectric elements into very small pieces to reduce grating lobes

sweep speed—the operator-adjustable spectral Doppler control that increases or decreases the number of heartbeats visualized on the spectral display

systole—the time period of the cardiac cycle when the heart is contracting

tachycardia—a heart rate that exceeds the normal rate for the age of the patient

tardus parvus—an arterial waveform shape with a delayed peak systolic upstroke that indicates proximal obstruction

temporal resolution—also known as frame rate, ability to display moving structures in real time

TGC—time-gain compensation; *see* key term compensation

thermal index—the calculation used to predict the maximum temperature elevation in tissues as a result of attenuation of sound

tissue Doppler imaging (TDI)—color Doppler imaging technique used to image wall motion

tissue harmonics—harmonic signal produced by the patient and is a multiple of the fundamental frequency; also referred to as native tissue harmonic imaging

tissue-equivalent phantom—the test object that mimics the acoustic properties of human tissue and is used to ensure proper equipment performance

total attenuation—the total amount of sound (in dB) that has been attenuated at a given depth

transducer—any device that converts one form of energy into another. May also refer to the part of the ultrasound machine that produces sound

transmural pressure—the pressure inside a vessel compared with the pressure outside of a vessel

transverse waves—type of wave in which the molecules in a medium vibrate at 90° to the direction of travel

triplex—the ability to visualize real-time grayscale, color Doppler, and spectral Doppler simultaneously

tungsten—component of the backing material

turbulent flow—chaotic, disorderly flow of blood

variance mode—the color Doppler scale with mean velocities displayed vertically on the scale and turbulence displayed horizontally

vasa vasorum—a network of small blood vessels that supply blood to the walls of arteries and veins

velocity mode—the color Doppler scale with mean velocities displayed vertically

vertical depth—the distance from the transducer

viscous energy—the energy loss caused by friction

voxel (volume element)—the smallest component of a 3D image

wall filter—the operator control that eliminates low-frequency, high-amplitude signals caused by wall or valve motion; also called high-pass filter

wavefront—the leading edge of a wave, formed as a result of Huygen's principle, which is perpendicular to the direction of the propagating wave

wavelength—the length of a single cycle of sound

wavelet—a small wave created as a result of Huygen's principle

write zoom—the type of magnification performed in the A-to-D converter (preprocessing) that magnifies the image by redrawing it before it is stored in memory

x-axis—the plane that is perpendicular to the beam path

y-axis—the plane that is parallel to the beam path

z-axis—the brightness, or amplitude, of the dots on the display

INDEX

Page numbers followed by *f* indicate figures and those followed by *t* indicate tables.